Discovering the Cause

and the

Cure for America's Health Care Crisis

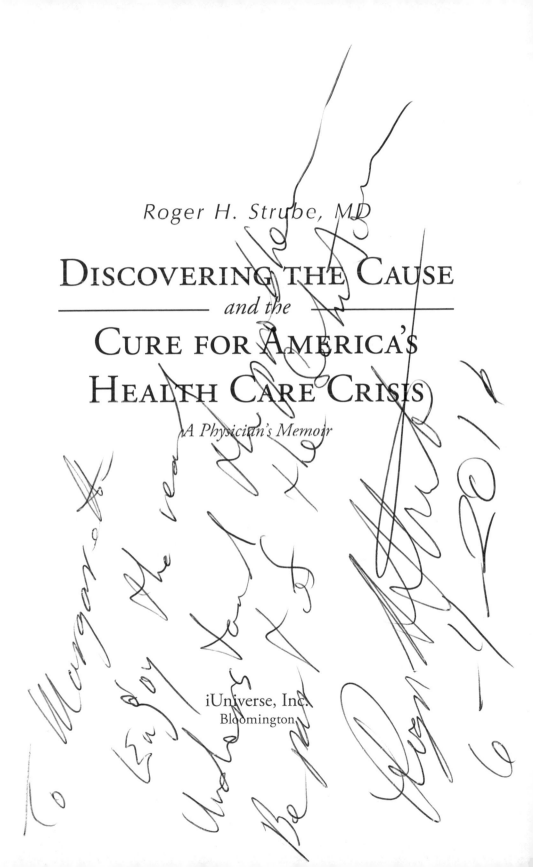

Roger H. Strube, MD

DISCOVERING THE CAUSE

and the

CURE FOR AMERICA'S HEALTH CARE CRISIS

A Physician's Memoir

iUniverse, Inc.
Bloomington

iUniverse books may be ordered through booksellers or by contacting:

iUniverse
1663 Liberty Drive
Bloomington, IN 47403
www.iuniverse.com
1-800-Authors (1-800-288-4677)

ISBN: 978-1-4620-0389-1 (pbk)
ISBN: 978-1-4620-0388-4 (cloth)
ISBN: 978-1-4620-0387-7 (ebk)

Library of Congress Control Number: 2011903662

Printed in the United States of America

iUniverse rev. date: 4/25/2011

Dedication:
For Kathy

Contents

Foreword

Roger and I are both sailors living in a boating community where sailing is more often the topic of conversation than are ruminations about careers, politics or sports. One memorable evening Roger and I sat on the aft deck of his boat, enjoying the sunset while anchored off a beach on the Southern tip of Florida. The sailing that day had been good. A fine dinner had been served, and now it was time to relish the evening and share stories and libation.

Done with tales of the sea, we began to talk about our past careers. Roger had been a primary care physician and the medical director for a number of HMOs. I had spent a career with what was the first Health Maintenance Organization (HMO) in New Hampshire—the Matthew Thornton Health Plan. Although ownership of the organization changed over the years, I remained and was for a long time one of the medical directors of the Health Plan and the Medical group, a part of Dartmouth-Hitchcock. Both of us had spent many years in the trenches of health care delivery. Roger had mostly been the medical director in one or another Preferred Provider Network—in other words, the doctors contracted with the HMO but were not employed by the HMO. Our group started as a staff model HMO—the HMO hired the providers as employees.

We discussed health care in America and, although we had both worked in different health care delivery models, we agreed that America's present system is too costly, unfair to many and ultimately unsustainable in its present form. Both of us had adopted the HMO concept early. We believed that it was a reasonable methodology of health care payment and delivery. Patients should be able to pay a fixed amount that assures the provision of necessary health care.

We agreed that there is no perfect system, but that we must find a better one. We discussed our conviction that a key element of health care should be the maintenance of health in contrast to a system that pays only for episodic care of illness and the treatment of unanticipated events. With the monetary incentives of the HMO structure, there are incentives to keep people healthy.

We are doctors who believe free enterprise solutions to most business ventures promote better outcomes through economic incentives.

My own group was founded on the premise that physicians should receive a salary rather than be paid for services. Our incentive was to keep the population under our care healthy, thereby decreasing the cost of care. Additional pay would come if the group as a whole did well. The local medical community initially shunned the first idealistic members of our group as Socialists and Communists. Although we were called "limousine liberals," we were clearly not part of the establishment. Most of us drove humble, inexpensive cars, and did not belong to country clubs. Our founder was staunchly Republican and economically quite conservative.

Many of us have become disillusioned about what HMOs can accomplish in recent decades. Over the years, many HMOs were transformed from organizations interested in promoting health by managing care to profit-centered megaliths that select healthier patients and deny needed care to improve their bottom lines. Many traded ideals for profit.

In this book, Roger shares his journey of discovery through organized medicine. He outlines the influences that formed his worldview of health care from early childhood through retirement. He describes many of the methodologies he instituted both as a doctor and as the director of an insurance company to promote better health. This book presents a mixture of life experience, philosophies, a polemic on heath care, and a description of what he feels works to keep people healthy.

Roger and I come from the traditions of process improvement where we find most errors are the results of system failures rather than individual folly or malevolence. We think it better to fix the problem rather than affix the blame. His often-repeated refrain that medical care is too frequently formed by memory-based information systems rather than from real data and tested guidelines is appropriate and accurate.

Further, many physicians bristle at the thought that the use of guidelines means abandoning principles of autonomy and training—what I call "cookbook" medicine. This harkens back to a fondly but inaccurately remembered era when it was possible for an individual to know all there was to know about medicine. The doctor's personal knowledge and experience were enough to make the best medical decision for that time and place. A competent physician could remember medicine's limited understanding of disease states and the few available cures. Today, research and development have greatly increased existing knowledge and resources tremendously, but no mere mortal could possibly contain it all in the confines of one brain.

Medical care has become too complex and, like pilots who rely on checklists to assure that established procedures and methods are followed, physicians should think of guidelines as an essential way to avoid error. Most serious and some deadly errors result from a cascade of events that usually start with a simple and avoidable event or action. Memory-based decisions too often leave out small steps thought to be insignificant that are ultimately critical. For example, remembering to order a mammography or colonoscopy can save lives, regardless of the reason that brought the patient to the doctor's office. System approaches, often assisted using electronic medical records, can help to avoid these omissions.

Roger and I have collectively worked over 60 years in the private sector. We understand the problems of our health care delivery system and we know there are no easy answers, but we see promise in the single payer system that other countries have adopted. Other industrialized countries that have chosen a single payer system certainly have problems in their health care systems. However, these systems seem to be working better on many fronts than the system now in place in this country. Consequently, we believe a single payer methodology is the best solution for American medical financing and care delivery problems. The choice to reform our funding system is difficult, but something must be done.

In an atmosphere of demagoguery, political posturing moves aside rational debate and "winning" becomes more important than good outcomes. Our country has refused to take the best from single payer systems and find ways to avoid the pitfalls. Instead, politicians emphasize the negatives without acknowledging the positives.

Universal health care financing will decrease costs for many patients, we acknowledge that it will increase some costs. We understand no change is possible that will not affect some group negatively. Many people forget that the unnecessary test, medicine, or surgical procedure performed on a patient is profit for some provider. Health care reform will increase revenue for some providers and decrease it for others, but we believe it will be a better allocation of resources on the overall balance sheet.

The Dartmouth Atlas of Health Care (www.dartmouthatlas.org) studies have shown that there is wide variation in cost and care in different parts of the country without demonstrably better outcomes.[1] Health care facilities are duplicated in small communities that do not need them. The Dartmouth Atlas presents clear evidence that greater volume leads to better outcomes. Centralization of many services would lead to better and less expensive health

---

1   See, for example, Regional and Racial Variation in Primary Care and the Quality of Care Among Medicare Beneficiaries (http://www. dartmouthatlas.org/downloads/reports/Primary_care_report_090910. pdf)

care. It is odd that we would drive half an hour for a pair of shoes on sale yet think it an imposition to have to drive as far to have a hip replaced, or to have heart surgery.

In a system without infinite resources (and there is no system where resources are expanding forever), tough choices must be made about how to utilize scarce resources. Money is the most relevant scarce resource for a large segment of the American population. America now rations health care based on economics. If you don't have a job, or you can't afford your own individual care, you live without adequate health insurance. An unexpected or critical need for care can disrupt your future. In 2001 medical causes accounted nearly 50 percent of families to declare bankruptcy, many of whom initially had insurance, were college educated, and had considered themselves securely in the middle class.[2] Appropriate use of resources—using medicines, procedures or methods with substantiated evidence-based outcomes—has been mislabeled as "rationing." A favorite method of any demagogue, re-defining the terms of the debate (such as equating end of life counseling with "Death Panels") has been a key method to muddy the waters and prevent useful, critical, productive discussions that might find a solution to the mess we're in.

The health care debate needs to focus on the increasing and unsustainable portion of the nation's GDP that our current system has engendered. A system motivated only by profit will do what is necessary to maximize income. Our health care financing industry attempts to control risk and maximize profit by covering healthy customers while for-profit insurance companies also limit or eliminate coverage for some who appear less healthy and thus more costly. Our medical delivery system increases profit by doing more tests and procedures that are sometimes unnecessary and ordering medicines of questionable value.

A single payer system does not mitigate all the problems in health care financing or health care delivery. Our present system rations health care based on the economics of the family. The single payer universal health care system eliminates economic rationing based on an individual's ability to pay for care. This financial reform would stop the single most important cause of bankruptcy in America: exorbitant and unnecessary medical expenses that most people cannot afford. It is our belief that the benefits of a single payer system far outweigh any downside.

---

2   MarketWatch: Illness And Injury As Contributors To Bankruptcy by David U. Himmelstein, Elizabeth Warren, Deborah Thorne, and Steffie Woolhandler. (2 February 2005). Retrieved on November 26, 2010 from http://content.healthaffairs.org/cgi/content/full/hlthaff.w5.63/DC1

There is no perfect system, There are only choices, some better than others.

To join the modern world, medicine must not equate high tech with greater value and high expense with better care. The illusion that all maladies can be cured must be abandoned. The healing arts must again be joined with science so that the caring physician will recall that where science ends empathy and sympathy must continue. Alleviating suffering is a value often more important than an illusory cure. Nevertheless, to the extent possible, our choices should be based on evidence rather than intuition, fact rather than hope.

In this book, we see one person's struggle to confront the issues of health care delivery, and medical resource management. Roger's experience can help all of us formulate informed decisions about health care delivery choices that confront us all both individually and as a group. His odyssey is one that can help us make informed decisions on all on these vital matters. Roger's life has ricocheted through many of the outposts of medical care; its retelling is a rich tale with useful information and insights that can help find better solutions. Everyone should read this book.

Wesley R. Wallace, M.D.
Medical Director Ret.
Dartmouth-Hitchcock Nashua NH
Dartmouth-Hitchcock Nashua NH

Preface

Walter Cronkite once said that America's health care system was neither healthy, caring, nor a system. Uncle Walt had it right. I have often wondered if American health care was ever any of these things. According to the Centers for Medicare and Medicaid Services, Office of the Actuary, National Health Statistics Group, our society dedicates 17.6 percent of the GDP or $2.5 trillion dollars[1] per annum to the medical-industrial complex. Over $8,000 per person is an extraordinary amount of money considering at the turn of the Millennium, the World Health Organization ranked the American health care system number thirty-seventh in the world. Since then, medical costs have skyrocketed and there is no reason to believe quality has improved.

This book presents an insider's perspective on health care delivery and financing. My experience with the health care industry spans thirty-six years of medical education, training, practice and administration. I practiced medicine for fifteen years before changing careers. My career in administrative health care continued an additional fifteen years. I am one of few people who have worked as both a family doctor and an insurance executive. I hope that my experiences and the conclusions I have drawn will help you understand why our medical-industrial complex is so costly and profoundly dysfunctional.

Activists and scholars produce megatons of wood pulp in the form of newspaper articles, Ph.D. dissertations, research studies, think tank reports, and books describing our health care crisis. The most notable and perhaps the best documented is the Dartmouth Atlas.[2] They all reach the same conclusion: the system is broken. Both the delivery of health care and the financing of health care delivery require reform.

If you believe our health care system is fouled up beyond all recognition

---

1   Centers for Medicare & Medicaid Services. "National Health Expenditure (NHE) Fact Sheet." Retrieved on January 18, 2011 from http://www.cms.gov/NationalHealthExpendData/25_NHE_Fact_Sheet.asp#TopOfPage.

2   For more details, see www.dartmouthatlas.org .

(FUBAR) but do not understand why or what can be done about it, you will find some answers in these pages. This book may be for you if:

- You are having difficulty separating reality from hyperbole about *health care insurance* and about quality *health care delivery.*
- You are confused about the health care financing approaches proposed and enacted by our federal government.
- You want to understand the potential unintended consequences triggered by insurance regulation reform.

This book is about my journey through our medical and insurance non-system. In some instances, I have used sarcasm and dark humor to point out problems we must address. The nurses, who have to deal with the flotsam and jetsam created by the anointed, may think to themselves, "It's about time someone pointed out our emperors have no clothes." We must understand what is broken if we are to fix our health care system.

Discovering the Cause and Cure for America's Health Care Crisis is not an academic term paper, destined to gather dust in some professor's library. It was written so the layperson might understand the causes of our crisis and enjoy the read if not the reality. My story builds understanding of our health care crisis incrementally. The tale, to the best of my memory, is real. In some cases I altered the names and places to protect the guilty. I have tried to limit personal stories to those with relevance. You would be correct in assuming that where I cannot remember the exact details I have made things up to put myself in the best possible light.

Discovering the Cause and Cure for America's Health Care Crisis is the story of the life experiences that helped to enlighten me and shaped my *Vision* of the future. This three-part memoir starts with my education and progresses through private medical practice into my administrative career, and explains my epiphany regarding the cause and cure for our health care system crisis.

My second book, *Creative Design for Health Care Reform,* offers more technical information for individuals interested in continuing the story to find out how we got into the mess we're in and how I think we should proceed to get us out of it. This second book is a must-read for staffers, politicians, health-care providers, and other policy- and decision-makers who might have the ability to actually do something about our health care quality and financing crises.

Many of the people in the medical-industrial complex have forgotten that we are here to serve our patients. Egregious profiteering, increasing the cost of labor to American business, has helped to precipitate our economic collapse. We are no longer competitive in the global economy. Thanks to Wall Street and other short-term thinkers, America is now experiencing a devastating economic crisis. Because of this crisis, this book is timely and urgently needed.

Health care reform is not simply a moral or social justice imperative. The debate about whether access to health care is a right or a privilege is important, but it is not the central focus of this book. As Bill Clinton said, "It's the economy, stupid." America is now several years into what economists may someday call the Second Great Depression. The excesses of Wall Street may have been the number one cause of our current economic devastation, but our health care system is certainly number two.

Only American business can pull our economy out of this depression. Business must control the cost of labor to remain competitive in the global market place and to get the economy growing again. Benefit packages, of which health care makes up the largest portion, are a major contributor to the cost of labor. The cost of health care must be reduced if America is to pull out of our economic depression. This is not a Democratic or Republican issue. It is an American issue.

Enjoy the read. When you are finished, please recommend the book to your doctor and your congressional representative. Your life may depend on it.

Acknowledgements

My experiences, observations and conclusions have occurred over a lifetime of interactions with tens of thousands of people. Overwhelmingly, these interactions were positive. As my father would say, "I've had a good run." Many of these folks helped me negotiate an interesting and satisfying personal and professional path and had a direct influence on the philosophy I express in this book. Most helped by simply encouraging my questioning mind. Counted among these are family, friends, teachers, and coworkers. Perhaps the most important group, my patients, put me on the path toward the light. A few of these supportive people are mentioned in this book but, obviously, naming everyone is impossible. How could they all be remembered? The human mind is not up to the task.

Two individuals stand at the core of my vision of our future reformed health care system. The first is Dr. W. Edwards Deming, the father of quality improvement. He was truly a beacon of light in a sea of mediocrity and darkness. The principles of continuous quality improvement and the management style he promoted still make good sense. His focus was business, but I could see the direct application to medical care.

The second individual is Dr. Lawrence L. Weed, the father of the problem-oriented electronic medical record (POEMR) and medical decision support tools. Exposure to his philosophy regarding decisions made by the unassisted human mind and the use of computers to medicine was a key lesson in what must happen to improve our medical system. The combination of Dr. Deming's continuous quality improvement (CQI) management philosophy and Dr. Weed's practical application of computers to some of the core problems in our health care delivery system formed the foundation for my vision of the future.

I must also acknowledge the part that the medical-industrial complex has served in motivating me to write this book, although it certainly deserves no thanks. Managed care, the vehicle to carry the vision forward, has been floundering as the American economy continues to support the excesses of the medical-industrial complex. No solution to any problem will succeed without a clear business need for its development and application. Unfortunately, the self-interest of many movers and shakers in American finance, housing industry, and health care system has put the economy into a death spiral, precipitating the need for reform.

When I started writing, my wife Kathy and I were anticipating our forty-sixth wedding anniversary. I thought the process would take six months. The economy continued to circle the drain for another two years as I wrote on. Kathy's ability to proofread the manuscript with a discerning eye has been most appreciated. Our daughter, Jill Strube Blasco, formed the other half of the home front tag team. Jill is the grant writer for the City of Smithville, Texas, and works part-time at the University of Texas in Austin editing papers for publication. The value of their technical support as editors and proofreaders was critical. Without their support and assistance, this book could not have been completed. Often, just as Emperor Joseph II reportedly said to Mozart regarding *The Abduction from the Seraglio*, "...there are too many notes," they would say to me, "Too many words." I did not reply, as Mozart would have, "There are just as many words as there should be." They made sure I did my best to stay on point. The reader will have to judge if they were successful.

I contacted many old friends and folks I worked with over the years to help more accurately document history. Some volunteered to do partial chapter proofreading. Charles Larson, one of my best high school friends and a retired marketing executive, helped simplify the Preface. Kristine Mogen, whose father originally worked out of my first solo practice office, was especially helpful in remembering the early years. Susan Giaimo and Michael Mihlbauer provided input about my early years of practice and volunteered meaningful editing time. Several coworkers from my first medical administrative positions provided historical information and volunteered editing time. These folks included Ed Elder, David Willis, Tom Lynch, Frank Fugiel, and Michael Bina. Helpful coworkers from later periods of employment include Randy Crenshaw, Michael Schaefer, Jerry Marsh, Gwen Cox and Mary Woolley. Lynda Bluestein filled in the gaps regarding my consulting gigs.

Mary Chupak, a retired English teacher and neighbor, volunteered many hours of proofreading time to correct my grammar, punctuation and spelling. My original teacher and part-time pre-school caregiver, Auntie Nancy Skrobis, participated in proofreading and with memories of the early years. She was also helpful in identifying when the writing became too technical for most readers. Dr. Wesley Wallace, the author of the Foreword, became a good friend when we moved to Punta Gorda. He is a retired orthopedic surgeon and prior medical director at a staff model HMO in New Hampshire. We had similar career paths and similar opinions regarding our medical-industrial complex experiences. His proofreading and input regarding the medical issues presented was invaluable.

Susan Montgomery, an old friend and professional medical editor and publisher, did the final suggestions and editing. Her knowledge of medical writing and publishing was well worth the cost of her professional services.

The folks at iUniverse, my online publisher, provided professional assistance in turning the manuscript into a book. Self-publishing and online publishing have come a very long way during the past ten years. Without their ability to fast track printing and marketing, the window of opportunity for this book to make a difference for patients and the American economy could have closed.

Finally, the American public and you, the reader, must be acknowledged. *Discovering the Cause and Cure for America's Health Care Crisis* is just a story and the vision of a more rational health care system is a fairy tale without your action. Our citizens and the officials we elect will determine if healthcare reform efforts develop working solutions to the healthcare and economic crisis. My challenge to you is this: read this book and become part of the solution.

PART ONE
Education and Medical Training
1947–1956

CHAPTER 1:
Public School Education

I grew up on the South Side of Milwaukee in an area called "Bay View" as America was coming out of the Great Depression. I was a child in the 1940s and 1950s as the working classes were rapidly rising to the middle, and our family was among them. My father's first job was for the Wisconsin Electric Power (WEP) Company at the Lakeside Power Plant, the first facility in the world to exclusively burn pulverized coal. The huge furnaces required periodic cleaning. My father was one of the workers that crawled into the fireboxes and, using a long metal rod, knocked the "clinkers" off the interior walls. The extreme heat and ash dust meant the workers had only a few minutes to clean out the furnaces and shovel out the ash before the fires had to be lit up again. During the 1930s and early 1940s minimal protection from breathing in ash and coal dust was available or required. He would come home with black clothes and a bad cough from his time in this inferno and quickly sought a way up and out.

My father was a very smart man, and although he completed high school, his family could not afford to send him on to school. He was pragmatic enough not to regret this fact of his life, and realistic enough to know the true value of a good education. When I was an infant, he missed a promotion at WEP that went to a man with two years of college. He took a job as a firefighter to deal with intermittent infernos, to enjoy a better quality of life, and to work in a field that would ensure that experience would make a difference when promotions were decided. He also made sure that my sister and I understood from an early age that education was the key to our ability to succeed in this life.

Our family lived on the second floor of a two-family dwelling called a "flat" in Milwaukee. Bay View is a dense residential area with these kinds of small flats and single-family bungalows. Many families, including mine, did not own a car. The electric streetcar that took my father to work was a block away. The corner grocery store was three blocks from home. All the necessities of modern life were close.

At the time, Milwaukee had an excellent school system. Trowbridge Grade School was a short four-block walk down quiet city streets lined with mature elm trees. My mother became well acquainted with my teachers and the principal during my first four years, since my teachers seemed to think I was a "difficult child." I was bored, and this challenged them in many ways. When I entered Kindergarten, I could add and subtract two-column numbers and read some words. My Aunt Nancy spent many hours as my preschool babysitter playing "teacher." I had experienced a personal "Head Start" program before there was such a public program.

Knowing how things in the world worked was very important to me. My questions may have been those of a child, but I always wanted an answer. "That's the way it is," or "because I said so" were never satisfactory responses. From the time I could ask questions, I questioned authority. But my teachers were not amused with my continual probing for answers and I met with severe consequences when I questioned their authority.

As a Milwaukee firefighter, the city provided my father Blue Cross of Wisconsin hospitalization insurance coverage. During World War II, Congress had passed wage and price control legislation but facilitated employee benefit package expansion by exempting health care insurance from taxation. Many employers, including the City of Milwaukee, offered health care coverage. Our family had no significant barrier to using the health care delivery system. Our physicians had no financial barrier to the care they decided to deliver. At least in this respect, these were the "good old days."

First Encounter with the Health Care System

My first encounter with health care came when I was in fifth grade. When I was ten, I was admitted to Milwaukee Children's Hospital where I was to receive the standard surgical procedure used at the time for a common medical condition that our family doctor had discovered. I remember everything with crystal clarity: the hospital room, the bed, the chipped white porcelain vessels and painted medical equipment, the terrazzo floors, the gurney ride as I was wheeled down the hall, the suspended white glass globe lights passing overhead, and the big overhead light in the stark operating room.

As I lay on the operating table, three doctors in surgical garb stood in the hall talking. Much later, I would understand that these men were probably the attending surgeon, a surgical resident and a medical student. They walked into the operating room and the older man told me they decided to cancel surgery. Instead, I would be given medication only. Standard care now includes both appropriate drugs and laparoscopic surgery, but this was unusual for the day.

For the next several months, I rode the streetcar downtown at regular intervals to receive a "shot." I am sure it was an early anabolic steroid and was possibly an animal-based derivative. I was probably part of an early experimental study to determine the effectiveness of the steroid for this condition.

My medical care occurred before the Nuremberg Trials condemned the Nazi's human experiments in their concentration camps and, before the U.S. government acknowledged and ended the Tuskegee Experiment that monitored the progression of syphilis and responses to medicines in uninformed black males. My treatment happened before Congress passed the Human Subject Protection legislation that established review boards and ethics standards, greatly affecting how investigators must treat human subjects in the study of medicine.

Nothing had stood in the way of my uninformed enrollment in a study of the effectiveness of anabolic steroids. As luck would have it, there were no complications from the condition or from the medication. I did not go into early puberty, end up five feet tall, or grow antlers.

When I was a child, I thought as a child—unaware of most anything that didn't concern me. During the last couple of years of grade school, my awareness of the world greatly expanded. Korean War movies were playing at the local cinemas. Movie Tone newsreels were shown between double features.

I was building plastic models of battleships, F86 Sabre Jets and cars. Between the Weekly Reader news magazine in school and newsreels at the picture show, current events were a part of life in the 1950s. I was aware of the anticommunist antics of Wisconsin Senator McCarthy and of the long-running conflict in French Indochina. During the spring of 1954, black and white newsreel films showed the fall of Dien Bien Phu to the "Commie Menace." These graphic images of the reality of war in the news reels were in stark contrast with the romanticized Hollywood version.

Doubting Thomas or Critical Thinker

This was also about the time I finished catechism class at Immaculate Conception parish in preparation for confirmation. Like many young teenagers, I was into pushing boundaries, and I was still questioning authority.

It was abundantly clear the nuns were not there to answer questions. Although one of the young priests, Father Hickey, was a good speaker and his Sunday sermons had some relevance, the rituals themselves seemed incomprehensible, the Mass being spoken in Latin. When the Archbishop came by to question the class regarding Church dogma, he found that everyone in the class had memorized the catechism and passed the examination.

The ritual of first communion and Confirmation followed shortly. We would all be "certified" Catholics. Throughout my formal education, especially during the years of medical school and training, I continued to experience this cycle of memorization, regurgitation and certification. I believe my early tendency toward being a Doubting Thomas developed into my preference for critical analysis and problem solving rather than reliance on certified expert opinion.

As a Milwaukee firefighter, my father (I called him "Pa") was not paid very well, as is the case today. Certainly they are not paid in proportion to the service they perform for their communities. As a result, many work part-time jobs to make ends meet. All the firefighters I ever met had advanced handyman, mechanical and automotive skills. Their chosen profession (maybe for the adrenalin rush) was firefighting, but any of these men (and they were all men at that time) could have worked in heavy construction, the building trades or auto repair.

There was always some "project" going on where firefighters were helping each other build or repair something. I hung out with Pa at many of these activities and learned much from these men as well as the blue-collar workers in my own family. My uncles had electric, carpentry, woodworking and automotive skills. I worked with them on some of their "side jobs" and many family projects. By the time I graduated from Trowbridge Grade School, I could do some rough carpentry, bend thin wall conduit, pull wire, hook up electrical outlets and fuse boxes, change points, plugs, and oil, and hot wire a car.

Enjoyment of the work involved was not the main reward. The real joy came from understanding how and why things worked. When the project was completed, the satisfaction was in a job well done, which, during the Eisenhower administration of the 1950s, was it's own reward. I suppose this is the essence of the "Midwest Work Ethic." We all wore "I Like Ike" buttons as a proud declaration of this strong ethic.

My eighth grade teacher had been my father's teacher twenty-six years earlier. My father and Miss Mages made sure I was on my best behavior and focused on my school work. Nevertheless, questioning authority and doubting expert opinion would remain both a blessing and a curse for the rest of my life. Upon graduation, our class book referred to me as "The boy with the constant why."

Bay View High School: August 1956 to June 1960

Following the morning assembly on the first day of school at Bay View High School in 1956, the administration presented us with a "Loyalty Oath" stating we were not now nor had we ever been members of any secret organization. I thought it might have something to do with McCarthy, but I was not sure, and, in any event, I did not like signing a document I did not completely understand. School administrators never explained why we had to sign this document to gain admission. However, since I never had been a member of a secret organization, questioning the reason for this requirement would cause an unnecessary hassle. I signed it. Soon afterwards, early civil rights organizations challenged the constitutionality of these oaths and won. School systems across the country eventually terminated these oaths.

During the spring of 1957, I began helping one of our neighbors refinish an old wooden Lightening centerboard sailboat. I learned to sail with this neighbor and joined South Shore Yacht Club (SSYC) as a Junior Member. SSYC membership was comprised of a cross section of the working class and professionals living in Bay View and on the south side of Milwaukee. At 15 years old, I observed that the people who seemed the most successful in terms of their status, their rewards and what they could give back to their communities were the skilled tradesmen, lawyers, doctors and dentists.

I believed I could be a good doctor and decided I would practice medicine on the south side of Milwaukee if I made the grade. I studied high school Latin in the belief that such knowledge would be required for advanced medical training. This turned out to be useful, but not necessary. My father, a Captain on the Milwaukee Fire Department, had always wanted me to be a Civil Engineer. This was understandable, since he had grown up during the First Great Depression and, because of Franklin Delano Roosevelt's Works Progress Administration (WPA) public works projects, the civil engineer was at the top of the "working man's" ladder. I was more interested in electrical "stuff" and if I had gone into engineering, it would have been in the electrical or electronics field.

The Space Race and the Importance of Education

These are the halcyon days in America that people want back. Getting it back is an impossible dream. Everything changed on October 4, 1957, when the Russians launched Sputnik. America could no longer sit on its post

World War II accomplishments. Being the dominant world superpower would demand a very large price. Ike had seen the German Autobahn and began construction on the American super highway system, the greatest American civil engineering project to date. Government had to get bigger if we were to maintain world dominance.

Upon entering the space race and turning to engineering for large scale public works projects, the federal government became very interested in, and supportive of, education. In the fall of 1958, the Milwaukee Public School System developed special advanced curricula in math, science, history and English. I believe these classes were the direct result of the Russian space program. I was one of the eight students in a class of over five hundred who qualified for all four classes. We were allowed admission to only two, and, at that point, I was not interested in being either a writer or history teacher, so I did not choose the accelerated classes in English and history. It took me years to develop an appreciation for writing and to become a student of history. At Bay View High School, I enjoyed math and science. Several of us were always at the top of the class in these subjects. Mrs. Case, our geometry teacher, was one of my favorites. I have never forgotten her saying, "All work and no play makes Jack."

I met my future wife, Kathy, in biology class the next year. I impressed her when I helped her dissect a frog. Our relationship took some time to develop, as her father did not allow Kathy to date during high school. "Going steady" would have been out of the question. We participated together in group activities but would not date until we were in our first year at the University of Wisconsin—Milwaukee.

The college prep courses at Bay View High School left little time for "elective" studies. Working under the assumption that some college courses would require formal reports, Typing became one of my few electives, although few typed reports were required before desktop computers were developed. These keyboard skills remained buried deep in my memory banks not to be called up again until 1992.

I had to work hard to master my studies in high school. Academics were part of the game of life. Test results determined my score. The more I learned, the better I could play the game. I did understand, however, that acquiring knowledge was more important than being good at a game. It is the essential foundation for understanding how things in the real world work. Knowledge and understanding of the basic principles underlying everything in the world around us is essential if we are to solve problems.

Academics were not my only interest in high school. I also played football and was on the swim and track teams. High school athletic programs are important in developing team spirit and a sense of sportsmanship and fair play. Individual sports, such as track and swimming, help develop an understanding of the time and effort required to excel at any endeavor.

The next years rolled on, summer for sailing, fall for football, swim team during the winter snows and track in spring. Spring weekends were spent sanding and painting boats in preparation for sailing during the summer.

Kathy and I graduated in the Bay View High School class of 1960 and registered for classes at the University of Wisconsin—Milwaukee. Following my eighteenth birthday in August of 1960, I registered for the draft and received a student deferment while attending the university. I was determined to strive for higher education and become a professional. I was not going to inherit a law firm, so I focused on working toward a medical degree.

If these goals did not work out, electrical engineering would be my failsafe, fallback final answer. Uncle Benny had one of the first transistor radios produced in the late 1950s, and I was very interested in electronics. As a Boy Scout, I had put together a "Crystal Radio" and built several Heathkit projects. I have often wondered where I would be now or what I would be doing if I had gone into electrical or electronic engineering at the dawn of the transistor and computer age.

The University of Wisconsin—Milwaukee: 1960 to 1964

Few people had noticed the official start of the Viet Nam War in 1959. The news reports of the communist threat and increased American presence in Viet Nam by the Democratic Administration sounded a muted far-away alarm. Current events were overcome by the pressures of studying and working our way through school, so I hardly took notice of President Eisenhower giving us the warning that "we must guard against the acquisition of unwarranted influence, whether sought or unsought, by military-industrial complex" in his farewell speech on January 17, 1961.

Kathy and I attended the University of Wisconsin—Milwaukee from 1960 to 1964. I use the term "attended" advisedly since we were commuters and never really had the "going away to college" experience. Our college grades suffered only minimally because of our need to work to pay tuition and living expenses. We are both from working-class families and although money was tight, our families valued education highly. We were the first generation in our families to enter any university.

Our parents viewed higher education as a training exercise similar to an apprenticeship. Achieving a college degree that would certify our qualifications to perform useful, well-paying work was the only goal they had for us. How could they understand that a college education is as much about training the mind in creative problem solving as it is about learning facts, passing tests and becoming certified. The concept that the college experience is a socialization process and a vehicle to make early contacts with others in our classes was unknown and unknowable to them.

We lived at home and worked our way through college. Kathy worked summers at Allen Bradley, a well-known Milwaukee light manufacturing employer where her father worked as a punch press operator. She also worked part-time as a cashier at one of the grocery stores in a local chain. I worked at a part-time evening job at Allen Bradley in the office doing parts and inventory control while I attended classes. In those days, the most sophisticated devices we used were "electric" calculators that had replaced the old, one-armed bandit mechanical version. The people on the evening shift who arrived at work a little early got the electric motor-driven mechanical calculators.

For anyone who has never seen or used such a device, the term "calculator" is an overstatement. They were actually simple mechanical adding machines that used an electric motor to drive the internal clockworks. They printed out the result of the addition on a long strip of paper similar to a grocery tally. These machines had no memory and, once the tallying was finished, these paper trails were buried in file cabinets with the stacks of invoices. Surprisingly, despite today's much more advanced technology, this is similar to what happens to many medical reports now.

During the summers, I was a Milwaukee County Park Commission Life Guard. I progressed to the position of Life Guard Supervisor for the pools and beaches on the South Side of Milwaukee by my final summer with the County.

Kathy studied education and became a grade school teacher. I focused on the pre-med curriculum and worked toward a Bachelor of Science Degree. The pre-med and Bachelor of Science curriculum were jammed tight with required courses. During my four years at the University, my schedule permitted time for only two elective class. I believed coasting through an Art or Music Appreciation course would not help gain acceptance to a medical school. Because mathematics is the basis for all science, I selected Calculus I and Calculus II.

One Christmas break prior to final examinations I was facing a time crunch and could not afford to take any time away from studying. My qualitative analysis chemistry instructor had assigned unknown chemical solutions to our class as part of the final exam. The University closed the lab over the holidays, so I would not have access to the necessary standard chemical testing solutions or equipment needed to determine the correct answer. Another student and I collected small quantities of all the chemicals needed to do the testing. His apartment had a gas outlet. We had a Bunsen burner, the small test tubes and other glassware necessary to process the unknowns. We did not have a centrifuge. Having had the interest in electronics and knowing how to make one came in very handy.

I had an old wire recorder motor attached to the original aluminum recording spool. (I never throw anything away.) I picked up a small aluminum cooking saucepan, removed the handle, and mounted the motor inside with the spool outside the bottom. A piece of spring steel strapping was bolted across the spool with each end bent down at the edge of the spool. Four inches further out each end was bent sharply up. A short nipple of brass pipe was attached to the spring steel on each side using a hose clamp. A small piece of foam rubber cut to fit filled the bottom of each pipe nipple so the test tubes would not fracture. Processing the unknown chemicals took several days. We submitted the correct answers and aced the course.

All that background in tinkering also helped with my Physiology course, which required a nerve conduction velocity experiment. I designed and built a Plexiglas chamber for the experiment. The chamber had humidity and temperature controls to keep the frog spinal cord, nerve and muscle preparation alive long enough to collect the data. I took the chamber with me for my medical school interviews. The project may have helped me secure medical school acceptance.

Science, Philosophy, Religion and Politics

The pre-med science courses took up most of my time in preparation to make a living, but the non-science courses have had the greatest impact on my political beliefs. The professor for the required Economics 101 course was an Adam Smith disciple and turned us all into aspiring capitalists, entrepreneurs and moderate Republicans. This would influence many of my decisions about how to take advantage of business opportunities and my propensity to vote for Republican candidates for most elections.

In contrast to those lessons in economics, the required anthropology course brought into focus the role superstition and religion play in primitive societies where natural phenomena are poorly understood. Primitive societies see gods in all things they do not understand. Our modern industrial science based society has explained much in our natural world. We no longer throw virgins into the volcano to appease the gods. Most modern religions speculate about our origins, provide guidance for our days on earth, and offer a comforting ideology about what happens to our individual consciousness when our bodies die.

My evolving understanding of the history of religion convinced me that conservative fundamentalist beliefs cannot be allowed to influence scientific research or the practice of medicine. Some religions profess to have a superior moral compass and attempt to use political power to force their beliefs on the rest of society. The last time this was successful, the world entered the Dark Ages. The Spanish Inquisition and many European wars followed. I am convinced that the mix of religion and politics makes a very toxic cocktail for the people. In Matthew 22:21 Jesus said, "Render unto Caesar the things which are Caesar's, and unto God the things that are God's." Our Founding Fathers may have had this passage in mind when they had the good sense to establish the separation of Church and State and guarantee our religious freedoms. That much I did get out of my American History class. Our Founding Fathers may have been iconoclasts.

Just as the Founding Fathers established the separation of Church and State to guarantee the widest range of freedoms for all, I believe that the Church should be separate from the business of medicine. Doctors and patients must make heart-wrenching decisions when an individual's health or life is in decline, and often find solace in their religion. However, basic human secular principles found in virtually all religions create the foundation for the Human Subject Protection legislation that requires certification of all medical, social, political science, and other researchers. However, I have seen too many cases of religion getting in the way of the practice of good medicine, more often as representatives of the Church attempt to wrestle power away from doctors, patients, and representatives in government.

I turned twenty-one at the end of the summer of 1963, just before entering my last year of undergraduate study. Wisconsin law defines the age of consent at eighteen for women and twenty-one for men. Kathy and I wanted to marry in June but several obstacles stood in the way. My father believed a man should be responsible for his decisions. He refused to sign the papers allowing us to be married any earlier than my twenty-first birthday. Kathy's family was Lutheran and I had been brought up Catholic. Her father was uncomfortable with the prospect of a mixed marriage. Much to the chagrin of Kathy's father, we were married as soon as parental permission was no longer needed. Kathy and I were married in the August before our senior year and prior to my application and acceptance to medical school.

During my senior year, I took the Medical College Admissions Test (M-CAT) and scored high enough to be considered for admission to several medical schools. Presentation of the physiology course nerve conduction velocity chamber at my medical school interviews may have secured my acceptance.

Although our families were learning to live together at this time and life was just beginning for my wife and I as a married couple, America was in turmoil and chaotic from the end of 1963 through the end of 1964. President Ngo Dinh Diem of South Viet Nam was arrested and assassinated in a military coup d'état backed by our CIA on November 2, 1963. Lee Harvey Oswald assassinated President John F. Kennedy on November 22, 1963. Most adults today remember where they were when they heard the announcement of his death. I was on a grassy knoll in Sheridan Park on a field trip, collecting plant specimens for a biology class assignment—one of the students was listening to music on a small portable radio when the broadcast was interrupted with the tragic news.

On August 7, 1964, Congress passed the Gulf of Tonkin Resolution authorizing President Johnson to use military force in Southeast Asia without a formal declaration of war. The Draft and whether Southeast Asian countries would fall, like dominos, to Communism were frequent topics of discussion. Because of the Draft lottery, eligible young men would have no choice about military service. I did not believe the Asian Domino Theory and was opposed to the war and the Draft.

Americans were split on the issue of Viet Nam. In my mind, there was no justification for our involvement in Southeast Asia. Most political satirists were against the war. George Carlin quipped we needed their rubber. When Curtis LeMay reportedly stated we could bomb North Viet Nam back into the stone age, Carlin observed that was worth about five minutes.

I voted for the Republican Barry Goldwater in the 1964 election. The majority of Americans wanted to continue the legacy of JFK. Lyndon B. Johnson won the election. The race to land a man on the moon and the Viet Nam war continued. As the war escalated and more troops were committed, the broken minds and bodies, and those in full metal jackets began coming home in greater numbers.

CHAPTER 2:
Private Medical Education and Training

In my senior year of undergraduate education at the University of Wisconsin–Milwaukee I applied to, and was accepted at the University of Wisconsin Medical School in Madison and Marquette Medical School in Milwaukee—both considered very good medical schools by medical professionals and the public alike. My choice was between what I perceived as a more academically-oriented medical education in Madison and a more clinically-oriented training in Milwaukee.

Because of my interest in practicing medicine in my community, I chose Marquette. There were several other reasons for making this choice. Kathy and I were married and both families and most of our friends and family lived on the south side of Milwaukee. Milwaukee was a much larger city than Madison with more opportunities for part-time and summer work for both of us to earn the money needed for tuition.

Marquette University is located just west of the Milwaukee downtown area on a small ridge overlooking the "industrial valley." One of the factories was the Ambrosia Chocolate Company and when the wind was right, the aroma of brewing chocolate would drift over the campus. The valley was also home to very large piles of coal used to produce power and heat for the city. The students could see these mountains of coal from some of the windows in the upper floors of the school.

The First Two Years

On a cool bright sunny day in September of 1964 Dr. John S. Hirschboeck, the Dean of the School of Medicine welcomed the Class of '68 to Marquette.

I do not remember any of the platitudes spoken that day, but I do remember the analogy he used regarding medical knowledge. He said we were facing the daunting task of studying and assimilating a vast amount of medical science. He likened the declarative knowledge we needed to the mountain of coal in the nearby valley.

The Dean said that our class was one of the most intelligent Marquette had ever admitted to the Medical School. He estimated our average IQ at 125. He had no doubt that our class was capable of shoveling through that great coal mountain of medical knowledge. He may have been shoveling something other than coal at us, but it seemed to make sense at the time.

Rev. W.H. McEvoy, S.J., who had a small coffee shop in the basement of Marquette Dental School, cared for the students' spiritual needs, helped alleviate their high stress levels and ministered to their soaring caffeine requirements. He was not only a man of profound faith but also a realist and a good man whom everyone liked and respected. Father Mac was a very down-to-earth Jesuit priest and never really "preached" or gave sermons to the students. I believe his mission was to bring back to the faith Catholic students who had fallen away from the Church because they had elected to embrace science.

He also believed that the guilt and shame regarding masturbation burned into the minds of Catholic boys had driven them away from the confessional and the Church. He once said, "The only boys who have never masturbated are the poor bastards born with no hands." I remember a convocation he held that first year where he focused on the fact that we were gifted but not special men (and two women) and our futures held the same pitfalls and limitations of all humanity. He predicted that some of us could fall by the wayside becoming drunks or addicts but that there could be a Nobel Prize winner among us. He encouraged all of us to try our best to be good physicians and good human beings; although the Nobel Prize winner has yet to be selected, his predictions were essentially correct—I think I am a good person and have been a good doctor, as have most of my classmates. I hope that Father Mac, wherever he is, believes I have reached these goals.

My daily commute to medical school took me over one of the long viaducts that spanned the industrial valley. Every day I looked at that mountain of coal and thought of the shoveling that was yet to be done. One thing troubled me as I looked down the industrial valley. There was always a long train of gondola cars bringing more coal to the mountains, just like the pile of medical journals arriving at the school library each month. The challenge seemed almost insurmountable.

On July 30, 1965 just after the end of my first year of medical school, President Lyndon B. Johnson signed the Social Security Act that created

Medicare. This event occurred as I was getting ready for my second year of medical school continuing to study that mountain of basic declarative scientific knowledge. Nationally, organized medicine opposed Medicare. The Milwaukee Medical Society, the American Medical Association and most of the practicing physicians I knew were opposed to the legislation fearing "government control and socialized medicine." Neither happened. It would be some time before I would know its impact on my career.

Medical school followed an educational model that was similar but much more intense than the usual college format. For two years, professors presented a massive amount of structured information by lecturing to large classrooms of students, assigning readings and administering tests. The professors organized this mountain of information into various related categories or epistemologies to facilitate teaching, studying and assimilating the most current knowledge.

Courses such as anatomy, histology, biochemistry, pharmacology and physiology provided the opportunity to study these disciplines in classes taught by professors who were experts with M.D. or Ph.D. degrees in each academic discipline. Some professors were better educators than others. Some were more entertaining than others. Some were more eccentric than others. Some were much more prepared than others. I remember very specifically one afternoon class when the professor arrived a little late, seemed somewhat disorganized and then, rather than launching into the lecture we expected, distributed a stack of "Blue Books." These are small blank page notebooks with blue covers used to administer essay exams.

It was obvious to everyone in the room that he was not prepared for the lecture he was supposed to give that day. He wrote on the board, "Contrast and compare Hodgkin's Disease and Malignant Lymphoma." We all put our heads down and started writing furiously. After about 20 seconds, one of my friends closed his Blue Book and walked to the front of the room where he dropped it on the professor's desk. When a group of us found him later in Father Mac's coffee house, we wanted to know what he had written. He said his answer was, "Hodgkin's disease is bad but Malignant Lymphoma is worse." Although this incident was never discussed in class, from that day on that professor was well prepared for all his lectures. We may not have been the smartest medical school class ever enrolled, but we were definitely among the most "smartassed."

I will never forget the year spent in the gross anatomy dissection laboratory. Spending time with the dead is one thing that sets doctors, morticians, and medical examiners apart from the rest of the world. To paraphrase a line I heard recently during an episode of a TV prime time crime drama, "The first day at medical school they give you a dead body to work on. That will change a person forever." It makes you more cynical, but also more serious. It brings you face-to-face with the finite nature of life and to a profound understanding that our short time upon this mortal coil is very precious. If there is a purpose to life, I believe it is to comfort and support our fellow human beings.

As a graduating class, we were very serious about our education and had a low tolerance for anyone who would waste our time. The students and the school had a large investment in our education. All knew that to reach our goals, we had to master a mountain of information. During these years, I learned more about the scientific method as applied to medicine and achieved a broad overview of medical science. Looking back, I realize we were just raking some coal off the surface, but had never truly made a dent in that huge mound.

The Clinical Years at Marquette Medical School

At the end of the first two years of attempting to shovel through this mountain of knowledge, I passed Part One of the National Boards of Medicine test and was allowed to progress into the clinical years of medical school. These were the days before all the federal oversight of pharmaceutical and durable medical equipment manufacturers. Eli Lilly and Company sponsored a weekend bus trip for our class and spouses, all expenses paid, to their manufacturing plant in Indianapolis, Indiana. The weekend included a tour of the facility and "scientific" presentations about their products.

At the time, this "educational grant" met the federal requirements regarding marketing products to physicians. Lilly is a major manufacturer of antibiotics and insulin, and a lot of good information using sound science was presented to our group. Everyone received a gift bag. This was not simply a bag of gifts. It was our first black "doctor bag" with gold embossed letters. Mine said, "Dr. Roger Strube" on one side and "Lilly" on the other. Inside was my first stethoscope also engraved with the word "Lilly." A small red rubber reflex hammer was included.

A special student discount had been arranged to purchase a Welch Allan Otoscope and Ophthalmoscope. There may have been several other shiny trinkets in the bag but I really do not remember. I had studied the basic medical science (declarative knowledge) and Phy Dog (procedures of physical diagnosis – procedural knowledge) but this first "Doctor Bag" contained the actual tools used to build one of the essential skills of practicing medicine – "Physical Examination." The gift reminded me of a Christmas long ago when my father gave me a small metal toolbox containing a hammer, pliers, two screwdrivers, a saw and a hand-operated drill.

The "educational seminar" and black bag built a sound relationship between the students and Lilly Company. They were very intentionally branding us and cultivating future relationships—a practice that ended as these relationships were found to develop brand loyalty that was sometimes stronger than the physician's objective determinations about the patient's need. This weekend was also memorable for the night at the "Rat Fink," a local nightclub, where I remember winning the belly-dancing contest (although I may be making that up).

During the clinical years of training, more declarative knowledge is acquired, and procedural knowledge acquisition begins to take on more momentum. During these last two years of medical school, I began to learn the hands-on techniques for doing minor procedures such as venipuncture (drawing blood) and suturing lacerations.

Marquette Medical School used several clinical locations in Milwaukee for educating students and training residents. Surgical and medical training was located at Milwaukee County General Hospital (MCGH) and Wood Veterans Hospital near the west end of Watertown Plank Road. The Woods Veterans Administration (V.A.) Hospital was much newer and meticulously maintained. It was a state-of-the-art facility at the time. County Hospital was much older and parts of it had been a tuberculosis sanitarium many years before. Woods V.A. was, after all, a federally funded facility and County General was funded by Milwaukee County.

These grounds were next to the Veterans Administration Domiciliary and grounds. Pediatric medicine and surgery were located at Milwaukee Children's Hospital, an old, disjointed building near downtown Milwaukee close to the Marquette campus. This organization has since become Children's Hospital of Wisconsin located on the main Froedtert Hospital campus. The study of Obstetrics and Gynecology happened at St. Joseph's Hospital on the north side of Milwaukee and at Milwaukee County General Hospital (MCGH, a.k.a. Froedtert).

The rotation through MCGH was very hands-on for medical students. The medical students had a great deal of latitude to order tests and medications, which were signed off by the senior licensed members of the team. The great majority of patients were the marginally employed, and unemployed, uninsured poor. Many were welfare recipients at the bottom of society's socio-economic and educational scale. They were essentially the poorest of the poor who had nowhere else to go for their care.

We saw patients with advanced, untreated breast, uterine and ovarian cancer. Some women had come in with septicemia, commonly called "blood poisoning," following botched back alleyway abortions. Several "obese" eighth and ninth grade girls seen in the emergency room for bellyache turned out to be in labor with unsuspected pregnancies. I remember walking past one of the delivery rooms where one of my classmates was attending the labor of a very large "grand multiparous" mother (a woman who has had many previous pregnancies). This was to be her fourteenth baby. She was on the delivery table, up in the stirrups, and Bob was standing between her ankles looking down as he adjusted his gloves. She let out one grunt and a ten-pound baby hit Bob in the stomach. Bob was quick enough to control the slippery lateral and the newborn did not slide out of his hands. All this happened in about a second and a half. We were literally "catching babies."

Most of these women were black, poor, and had no preadmission or prenatal care. Family planning services were at a minimum. Although Lyndon B. Johnson had signed the Social Security Act of 1965 into law on August 7, creating Medicare, the majority of our clinic patients were uninsured. Medicare did not reach most of these folks for many years. Roe v. Wade would not be decided until January 22, 1973. America's underclass and uninsured population was growing exponentially. I did not know it at the time, but these patients were the tip of the health insurance iceberg that our Ship of State has now impacted.

After MCGH, our internships took us to St. Joseph's Obstetrical service. Rotations through St. Joe's rolled through forty-eight hour shifts. Students spent thirty-four hours on call each forty-eight hours. Each on call shift started at 0800 on day one and carried through 1800 hours on day two. This was followed by fourteen hours off starting at1800 hours on day two through 0800 hours on day three. This schedule repeated every two days.

The contrast between MCGH and St. Joe's was sharp. Where the County's patients had been from the bottom of the socio-economic scale, the patients at St. Joe's were from the middle and upper class. The students at the St. Joe's rotation had no responsibilities other than to provide an admission history and physical (if the patient agreed to talk to the medical student) that was checked and signed off by the senior residents. The students were there simply to observe the care provided by the senior staff and study the literature.

This sounded like an easy rotation in comparison to MCGH, but it wasn't. Jack Klieger, M.D., Professor of Obstetrics and Gynecology at St. Joe's, insisted that all residents and medical students stay awake for the entire thirty-four hour shift. Residents and medical students had to attend patients or read obstetrics literature during their shift. Anyone caught napping was discharged from his service. This was a very rough rotation for me. During my every other night off I worked as a part-time first aid attendant at one of the local industrial plants. If no one came in for a band-aid or aspirin, I could sleep on a folding cot most of the night, but this wasn't always the case and to say I was frequently sleep-deprived is an understatement.

Things are now very different, as studies have shown that sleep deprivation interferes with concentration and learning. Enlightened minds have prevailed regarding the impairment of critical decision making and learning caused by lack of sleep, which has a devastating effect on coordination and the ability to perform complex tasks. A sleep-deprived physician may perform at the same level as drunken doctor. Fortunately, this boot camp approach to medical training has largely been abandoned.

It is one thing to study the circulatory system in textbooks followed by anatomy class where an embalmed body is dissembled. It is quite another to dress in blue pajamas, tie on a surgical mask, scrub, glove and enter the emergency room with a needle holder in hand to sew up a simple skin laceration. We practiced laceration repair using bare hands to sew up a piece of sliced foam rubber. (Another of the medical supply manufacturers provided the practice suture sets. These companies manufacture silk, catgut, or synthetic threads with swaged-on needles for all sorts of special situations.) Actually repairing a laceration on a human body with gloves on was much more difficult.

One of the surgical residents would have examined the injured patient to determine if anything important had been nicked. They were always looking for special cases, such as partially lacerated or severed tendons, deep lacerations or facial lacerations, to repair to build their surgical resumes. Residents log their cases so a record of experience may be documented. These logs are an example of the information hospital staffs or fellowship programs need for credentialing and vetting applicants.

A few renegade third and fourth year residents occasionally cruised the Veterans Administration Domiciliary (a.k.a., "The Dom") looking for potential elective cases such as hernia repairs. They needed to supplement the random distribution of surgical "cases" entering the emergency room.

An orthopedic resident I knew on a sixty-bed ward at the V.A. had an opposite problem. He was trying to improve efficiency by discharging patients when they were ready to go home. As a result, the ward usually had open beds and a higher turnover rate. This is very good for the owner and servers in a restaurant but not so good for the V.A. Professional Admissions Officer. V.A. hospitals were funded by the number of beds *occupied* not the number of patients treated and discharged. The Chief Resident with double-digit empty beds stood out like a sore thumb.

The old adage, "No good deed goes unpunished" was operative here. He learned that his efficiency would be rewarded with assignment to a ward filled with non-surgical cases. The Professional Admissions Officer would do what it would take to meet the metrics and maintain his funding. The residents soon learned to game "the system." The chief resident maintained either a full ward or fewer than ten open beds by using an unofficial short list of easily dischargeable patients. If a patient presented needing a surgical procedure, the patient would be admitted and one of the vets in the on deck circle would be discharged. The open bed counts and occupancy statistics remained stable. How is this different from full time workers in a union shop telling the part-time college kid working efficiently that he is spoiling their piecework compensation "rate?"

The Silver Stallion Meets Omentum and Other Early Lessons

While on rotation at Woods V.A. Hospital, one of the second-year surgical residents and I were on duty in the outpatient clinic. One of the older disabled vets (at that time, I considered people in their early 60s "older" – now, not so much) had a complaint of rectal bleeding. Rectal exam and a stool test did show the presence of blood. The anoscope, a short stainless steel tube, allowed visualization of large hemorrhoids but no signs of recent bleeding. A proctoscopy was scheduled and the man came back for the procedure several days later.

The patient was very apprehensive and "twitchy." The colon may be cut (biopsied) or burned (cauterized) without producing pain, but regardless, stretching the wall produces what some physicians refer to as "discomfort." As the resident advanced the rigid stainless steel proctoscope ("The Silver Stallion") just past half way and into one of the bends in the lower colon, the patient "whooped," lurched and then settled down—his colon had been punctured. The resident motioned me over to look in the scope. I saw yellow globules of fat. "Omentum?" I asked. "Yes" he replied. I asked, "Do you want to leave the scope in so we can find the hole?" He thought it would be easy enough to find since it was on the anterior surface of the bowel.

An operating room was open and the patient was taken to surgery. I scrubbed in for the repair of the torn lower section of the large bowel. The vet recovered without incident. No cancer was found, just internal hemorrhoids (very common in old alcoholics with cirrhosis). Clearly, the diagnostic test was indicated and necessary. The V.A. is not a fee-for-service (FFS) environment, so there was no perverse profit incentive for the resident. Perforation is a not uncommon complication of this procedure and a certain "acceptable" number of bad outcomes like this are anticipated. The resident was skilled in the procedure and careful in performance, but shit happens, especially during colon exams.

There is an anticipated level of risk of a complication with any invasive procedure or medication. Just listen to the T.V. ads for all the "Ask Your Doctor" medications. I hope that for any procedure or drug, the benefit to the patient is much greater than the risk. Consider procedures or medications that are not medically necessary and that have little or no benefit to the patient. Is it possible to establish an acceptable complication rate for unnecessary medical care and procedures? This key question is still relevant in health care reform discussions today.

The students at County General had more latitude and responsibility in caring for patients. Once the on-call surgical resident determined the adult patient had an uncomplicated skin laceration in an unimportant place (in other words, plastic repair would not be necessary), the medical students were allowed to do a single layer skin closure. These were the days of "see one, do one, teach one" and many third year medical students (MS3s) learned to stitch watching a fourth year medical student (MS4) do one.

The long journeys ending with board certification in any surgical specialty begin with these first steps, which included declarative and procedural knowledge education followed by physical skill training through doing the procedures repeatedly. At the same time, significant life-long relationship building between the physicians-in-training and the representatives of the medical supplier and pharmaceutical manufacturers was going on. Drug fairs were held in the medical lounges where pharmaceutical representatives would talk to the students, interns and residents about the newest advances in their products. Donuts, cookies and coffee were usually involved.

The instrument manufacturers would demonstrate their tools to the residents and staff. In some cases, these reps were certified surgical assistants who would actually assist in surgery in order to demonstrate the use of the new tools. Replacement parts manufacturers would display the latest in Teflon coated surgical stainless steel or titanium hips, knees, shoulders, and elbows. They also had qualified people to assist the surgeons with replacement procedures. American education and free market capitalism—what a combination, what a country!

During rotations through the last two years of medical school, I enjoyed orthopedics and radiology the most. This was probably due to my love for woodworking and tools. The biggest difference between woodworking and orthopedic surgery is that with woodworking, the artisan must be very precise and nobody dies. With orthopedic surgery, the surgeon has only to get the broken parts close and the bones will generally grow back together. My orthopedic professor once said, regarding an eight-year-old with a clavicular fracture (broken collarbone), if the two pieces were in the same room they would heal together. I knew I could be much more precise than that.

During my pediatric rotation at Milwaukee Children's Hospital, I took part in gathering data for the ongoing study of lead levels (Plumbism) found in children living in the old homes in the city core. This was the only time during my medical training that I directly participated in the "scientific method." The grunt work of gathering data was my only exposure. Statistical analytical training was not part of the exercise. I imagine the school administrators, curriculum planners and professors assumed that if you read enough scientific articles you would somehow gain an understanding of statistics as well as the medical information being presented. I remember one of the TV comics of the time saying, "Well I'm not a real doctor, but I hung around a drug store a lot!"

On November 9, 1967, Lance Sijan, one of my high school friends and a graduate of the Air Force Academy, ejected from his damaged F-4C over North Viet Nam by a fuse malfunction and premature detonation of a dropped bomb. Our military listed Lance as Missing in Action (MIA) until the North Viet Nam government confirmed he had died January 22, 1968. He was awarded the Medal of Honor posthumously on March 4, 1976. One of the Air Force Academy Cadet Residence Halls is named after him. Had he lived, I believe he would have been the Republican candidate for president in one of the past three national elections. A President Lance Sijan might have appointed me Surgeon General.

The Snow Storm, the Tavern, and the Ambulance

Nineteen sixty-eight started out very well for my family. On January 4, 1968, our daughter Jill was born at Trinity Hospital in Cudahy, Wisconsin, a suburb just south of Milwaukee. It was the middle of winter and my senior year in medical school. A snowstorm had hit the state as my wife went into labor. The electric power and phones at our house were out. Our cars were bargain-priced ten-plus-years-old, hand-me-downs from relatives. Snowdrifts surrounded both, but that mattered little, as neither would start.

The town ambulance was in a firehouse located about a half mile away. A tavern on the route was much closer. Milwaukee County has an excess of corner taverns. If they had power and a working phone, I would call the ambulance. If not, I could walk to the firehouse within twenty minutes. I walked several blocks to a tavern. Yes, I did say walked. There was no need to run. I knew that labor for primiparous mothers (first pregnancies) took in excess of 14 hours.

As I rounded the corner at the end of our street, the neon Schlitz Beer sign in a small tavern window lit the driving snow. I knew they had power. The phone worked and I called the fire department. The firehouse was about a quarter mile past the tavern. They would send an ambulance. As I walked back through the snow the ambulance passed me and was at the house when

I arrived. From the look the paramedics gave me, I knew Kathy had told them I went to the tavern when she went into labor.

The ambulance transported us to Trinity Hospital. This Cudahy hospital is now part of the Aurora Health Care System based in Milwaukee and named Aurora St. Luke's South Shore. I was in the delivery room when Jill was born and cut the umbilical cord. Back in those days new mothers stayed in "confinement" for several days. Bed days were relatively inexpensive back then, and this was probably done to give mothers with other children at home a break. The economics of the extended stays were not important; however, many children lost their mothers unnecessarily. Over time, medical studies found that the longer the new mother stayed in bed, the greater the chance of thromboembolism, a potentially fatal condition that occurs when blood clots in the legs break loose, pass through the heart and lodge in the lungs. The snowstorm passed and Kathy came home on the third day after giving birth.

Interestingly, studies have shown that the new mother is stable at about eight hours postpartum. Extended stays produce a great deal of expense, increased risk of thrombi and exposure to hospital-based infections. Although the clinical epidemiology (medical science) backed the eight-hour stay for the mother, the public, many physicians and all politicians were horrified at this recommendation. The only public health justification for any stay longer than eight hours after a normal, uncomplicated delivery is so the newborn may have the urine tested for phenylketonuria (PKU), a serious childhood disease. This is a simple test on a wet diaper easily preformed at home by a visiting nurse, lab tech or one of the parents. However, many physicians, all politicians, and most hospital administrators do not think their patients/constituents are bright enough or conscientious enough to perform the testing.

There may be some justification for their concern. If testing a child with this enzyme disease is missed, retardation may result. More advanced quality-oriented health care systems, especially Health Maintenance Organizations, developed the facility to send out home care nurses to check on the mother and newborn shortly after discharge. Much better psychological support and quality of care resulted. Unfortunately, as was the case with many HMO quality improvement programs, most of the public neither understood nor tolerated such quality improvement efforts, and couldn't understand how sending a home care nurse could possibly be more cost effective than keeping the mothers an extra day at the hospital. The politicians, physicians and hospital administrators soon joined the cause against this scientifically established cost-effective best practice.

The managed care organizations countered by contracting for a bundled fee for the mother and new bundle of joy. In lay terms, the contract stated,

"Kids stay free at Our Lady of Perpetual Profit Hospital." These contracts covered all uncomplicated deliveries and included C-sections for the same global fee so there would be no financial incentive for excessive length of stay or for doing unnecessary surgery. The financial policies had begun to move toward alignment with sound science.

At the turn of the last century hospitals were places where infections ran wild and people went to die. Much of the carnage was due to poor hygiene (i.e., poor sterile techniques and lack of repetitive hand washing). Separate facilities were built for "confinement" for childbirth. Early on, proposals were made to burn down the wooden structures every five years or so, to stop the ever-increasing infection rates.

The perception that hospitals were places where people went to die did not change significantly until after World War II and the use of Sulfa and Penicillin dramatically decreased infection rates. Unfortunately, the success of these drugs has resulted in the overuse of several generations of antibiotics, especially broad spectrum super drugs. Driven by physician over-prescribing and patient demand, "super bugs" resistant to all known drugs have evolved. Methicillin-resistant Staphylococcus Aureus (MRSA) is one such organism. Infections with these bacteria are usually hospital-based (nosocomial) and spread by poor sterile techniques, including inadequate hand washing. Infections from these organisms produce a high mortality rate. We may have to come back to providing special places for childbirth as a normal function of medical care. As medical care costs and complication rates have skyrocketed, more and more families have discovered birthing centers.

Nineteen sixty-eight was to be a year of tumult and rage for America. On January 30, 1968, the Tet Offensive began in South Viet Nam and resulted in over 15,000 Allied casualties. Walter Cronkite, Uncle Walt, the most trusted man in America, broadcast that the War was not winnable. LBJ realized if he has lost Cronkite, he has lost support of Middle America. On April, 4, 1968, Martin Luther King was assassinated at the Lorraine Motel in Memphis, Tennessee. On May 10, 1968, peace talks began between the United States and the Democratic Republic of Vietnam. On June 5, 1968, Robert F. Kennedy was assassinated in the Ambassador Hotel in Los Angeles California. From August 26-29, 1968, the Democratic National Convention was held at the International Amphitheatre in Chicago, Illinois. The antiwar protests in the convention hall and riots in the streets were broadcast live, around the world.

Internship—The First Half

Following the clinical rotations of the last two years of medical school, I took Part Two of the National Board Examination. All but a couple of people in the Marquette Medical School Class of 1968 passed Part Two and graduated with their "M.D." degree. The class of 1968 had two drop-outs and one suicide. Those of us who survived medical school and passed Part Two of the National Boards went on to a rotating internship and/or residency.

Most of my medical school classmates were nervous about Vietnam and the draft. Many had registered for an additional military draft deferment known as the "Berry Plan." Some believed they had a better chance of acceptance into the residency of their choice if the program administrators could be assured they would not be drafted out of training, which would mean leaving an open position. I had only taken one deferment for attending college and was eligible for the draft during medical school. The Vietnam War had been raging with increasing intensity through 1968, and the Democratic Convention had shown the United States to be at the point of open rebellion. Peace talks had started and Richard Nixon had made a campaign promise to end the War. I took the risk and did not apply for further deferment or the Berry Plan, believing all branches of the military would have more general physicians and specialists than they needed. This turned out to be an accurate read of the situation.

During these last two years of clinical rotations, medical students discover the next mountain ranges of knowledge they need to accumulate. Some graduate programs offered specialty residency programs that rolled this first year (internship) into the overall four or five years of postgraduate training. The first life-path decision is between the broad categories of Medicine and Surgery. During the senior year of medical school, the student decides which medical or surgical specialty to pursue. An application for an internship in a private or academic hospital that provides the best track toward that goal is submitted. If a specific specialty is not determined, many graduate doctors apply for rotating internships lasting one year.

Because I had become interested in Orthopedic Surgery and Radiology, I chose a rotating internship at St Luke's Hospital (now part of Aurora Health Care System), one of the largest and best hospitals in the Milwaukee area with a strong Radiology residency program and a heavy operating room schedule of orthopedic surgery. I was twenty-six years old just after starting my rotating internship. St. Luke's Hospital was also one of the leading hospitals for cardiology and cardiovascular surgery. It was located on the south side of Milwaukee twenty minutes from our home. The first half of my internship was very busy and very interesting.

The program director assigned the interns to community-based staff physicians. The intern worked under the direct supervision of this licensed mentor. The attending staff doctor would admit a patient. The licensed physician provided a working diagnosis and initial admission orders. The intern would see all admissions, and dictate a patient admission history and physical examination report. The admitting staff physician would also discuss the medical issues and plan for diagnosis and treatment with the intern. The mentoring physician would discuss all medical exams, notes and orders written by the intern. Any orders written by the intern were reviewed, discussed and, if found appropriate, countersigned.

The mentoring physician theoretically brought experience, medical skill and a warm bedside manner to the relationship. The intern, fresh out of medical school, theoretically brought the latest in medical science. In the greater scheme of education and training, this collaboration was widely believed to bridge the gap between the newest/latest in basic medical science and the wisdom/experience of the practicing physician.

Looking back, I believe there was much more downloading of bad habits than uploading of innovative thought or technology. Sometimes in this exchange of knowledge between the professionals focusing on the "case," the patient, as a unique person, is lost. Medical personnel all too often focus on the disease, losing sight of the human being. Many times this does not matter in terms of the outcome. In fact, it probably does not matter. The patient's disease, wants, needs, desires, and psychosocial make-up many times align with what the medical professionals perceive as the problem set and what the physicians are prepared to deliver in the way of care.

If everyone involved is on the same page, the patient and family will accept a predicted outcome, even if it is bad. There are times when nothing can be done for terminal patients but give them as much comfort, both medical and psychological, as possible. Sometimes things go badly or complications arise causing the outcome to be worse than expected. As long as everyone is well informed, most people will accept the result when unexpected bad outcomes happen.

There are times when problems and diagnoses are well defined and understood by all, but several plans of treatment with variable expected outcomes are available. The psychosocial situation and the desires, wants and needs of the patient then become paramount. The medical personnel will push for the plan that, in their view, offers the best outcome. Nevertheless, the patient must own the decision regarding the option chosen or, if the patient is unable to decide, the patient's designated family members must own the decision.

Treatment of prostate cancer typically falls squarely into this category.

Baring unusual circumstances, this disease comes with a thirty-year survival expectation regardless of how it is treated. During routine autopsies performed on men who have died of unrelated causes, fifty percent have undiagnosed prostate cancer. Early diagnosis may have little impact on real life expectancy. Depending on the situation, "watchful waiting" may have the same outcome, without all the complications of aggressive interventions.

Once the diagnosis is made, the treatment offered has more to do with the credentials and certifications of the doctor than the unique situation. The urological surgeon will usually want to cut it out. The radiological oncologist may want to zap it with radiation. The internal medicine physician trained in oncology will typically want to poison it. The endocrinologist will usually want to inject hormones. Patients must understand the problems and complications that are likely to occur with each proposed treatment and choose the plan that best fits their situation and their constitution. Keep in mind that when diverse experts offer very different therapies for a unique problem, none of the recommendations are exceptionally effective. It is not unreasonable for some folks to avoid all the complications of aggressive therapy by selecting "watchful waiting," especially for a diagnosis for something like prostate cancer.

Such reasoned decisions made in the bright light of informed consent are understandable. A decision to refuse active treatment and enter Hospice for supportive care and comfort measures made by a person of any age with a terminal condition within the last six months of life is not only acceptable and reasonable—in most cases it is the logical course to choose. A decision by a patient with no chronic terminal illness to refuse available standard care for a sudden life threatening emergency problem is illogical, unacceptable and repugnant to the physician proposing treatment.

The most frustrating patient I encountered during my year of internship was an otherwise healthy mid-20s mother of two small children with a massive gastro-intestinal bleed who had been transported to the hospital by ambulance. This young mother was bleeding to death. She agreed to the ordered diagnostic blood testing and the type and cross match of four units of blood. Although the testing was acceptable, she would not consent to the transfusions because of her religion. Emergency surgery was out of the question because she was so bled out she would not have survived. No surgeon would touch her without consent for the blood transfusions.

She was aware that without the transfusions she would die. However, logic failed and superstition prevailed. I consulted corporate counsel for the hospital and my staff advisor. If she had been under 18, we could have conceivably gotten a court order for the transfusions, but she was an adult, and we probably did not have time. The simple, established technology was ready for application at a moment's notice. I knew what had to be done and felt it was an easy solution with few possible physical complications, but there was nothing I could do to save her life.

We administered supportive care through the evening. She lapsed into a coma before midnight. Her large family, including her husband and two small children, prayed at her bedside all night. She died early in the morning, leaving her husband a widower and her children without a mother. My frustration with this family's religious fundamentalism was immense, but freedom of religion is a right for all Americans. Suicide by the refusal of standard emergency care also appears to be a right. A Presbyterian friend of mine told me his religion believed in predetermination and that God had a plan for everyone, but he still looked both ways before crossing the street.

Our Founding Fathers understood the dangers of a theocracy and state-sponsored religion. The first amendment to the Bill of Rights states, "Congress shall make no law respecting an establishment of religion, or prohibiting the free exercise thereof." I interpret this to guarantee "freedom from religion" as well as "freedom of religion." As frustrated as I was with her decision, this mother had a right to choose suicide (although she would not have framed it that way). But followers of her religious sect cannot be allowed to gain the political power to force their dogma on all other Americans. The right to choose how we live and how we care for ourselves must be protected.

I have learned from this and other personal experiences as a physician that there is a palpable danger to these freedoms for all Americans if right wing religious fundamentalists take control of and pull the levers of political power. As our country struggles to reform its medical care delivery system, Americans cannot allow religion and superstition to supersede science in determining what care is effective and medically necessary. We cannot allow religious extremists to determine the benefits of a national health insurance program or determine the exclusions or restrictions. Senator Daschle had many things right in his book, *Critical*.[1] One of the most important is the concept of taking politics out of the system by establishing a Federal Health Board that would determine standardized medical science criteria regarding what works. Only then may we determine a reasoned benefit structure, regarding what appropriate, effective and efficient care should be covered.

As an intern, I spent a great deal of time with one of our more active orthopedic surgeons whom I'll refer to as E.K. My duties included performing a complete medical history and physical (H and P) and dictating the report.

---

1   Senator Tom Daschle with Scott S. Greenberger and Jeanne M. Lambrew. (2008)., Critical: What we can do about the health-care crisis. NY: St. Martins Press.

An admission note and admission orders had to be written and posted on the chart or the patient would not be allowed entry to the operating rooms. The hospital staff rules required a completed H and P filed in the chart prior to all but emergency surgery.

Orthopedic surgeons understand pain management but are notorious for knowing very little general medical pharmacology. They usually obtain a "clearing consult" from an internist who writes the admission medication orders. The surgeon writes the pre-op and surgical orders. When I worked with an orthopedic surgeon, he would simply tell me to see the patient and write orders for some "herbs," what they called the drugs that managed the pain.

Scrubbing in with E.K. was a real treat. He was an excellent technical surgeon and knew anatomy well. I assisted with several laminectomies (back surgery for ruptured disk). After opening and exposing the lamina, E.K. would remove some bone and I would gently retract the nerve as he removed the ruptured disk. His patients did very well.

The Hard Working, Beer Drinking Alcoholic

One case I remember well had an excellent technical result but a near-disastrous outcome. A blue-collar worker in his early 40s entered the emergency room with an unstable fractured elbow after falling at work. All Wisconsin physicians loved to treat worker's compensation cases since payment was facilitated by the obligatory ambulance chaser. In addition, because the patient received disability pay until released for work, there was never any pressure from the patient or family to be released before the injury had healed, allowing for the best possible outcomes for the patient in most cases.

This patient had a family doctor who admitted him and consulted E.K. for surgery. His elbow was wrapped and iced and pre-op laboratory and X-ray studies ordered. The family doctor made rounds the evening of admission and dictated the pre-op medical history and physical examination. In the morning, review of the lab reports and X-rays were unremarkable except for the fractured elbow. I scrubbed in with E.K. for this apparently very simple, uncomplicated internal repair (screwing a shiny metal plate over the two pieces of bone to keep them in alignment).

The procedure was technically perfect and completed in a matter of minutes. However, not all was well. In the recovery room, the patient became responsive reasonably quickly but remained groggy. He was transported to his room where he seemingly became more alert but did not recognize his wife. He was alert and responsive but remained disoriented about time, place and person. A short discussion with his wife revealed that his history of "a couple of beers a day" was actually more than a case (24 bottles). Because of alcohol withdrawal and the stress of anesthesia and surgery, he had developed full-blown delirium tremens. Delirium tremens (DTs) has a 5 to 10 percent mortality rate if treated and up to a 35 percent mortality rate if untreated.

This patient was not like the alcoholics I had seen at Woods V.A. Hospital. The old, malnourished veterans had a typical body shape of muscle wasting in the arms and legs with a protuberant abdomen. They would get up in the morning and walk from the Domiciliary to one of the bars across the street. Because their hands shook so much before their first drink, they were not able to bring a glass of any liquid to their lips.

The veteran would order a beer in a can and a shot of brandy. The bartender would pour out a little beer and dump the shot of brandy into the can. The small holes in the top of the can limited spillage. The tremors did not prevent them from getting this fortified drink to their lips. After a few minutes, the shakes would stop, and they would be able to start some serious drinking for the day. As the old saying goes, "You cannot drink all day if you don't start in the morning." If one of these vets needed surgery, the residents at the VA would start DT prevention treatment on admission.

Our patient with the broken elbow was different. He was a well-nourished, hard working, hard drinking, blue-collar guy who had never missed a day of work. He was a Milwaukeean. He did not "look like" an alcoholic. He looked like a reasonably healthy forty-something working man with a broken elbow. The basic premise in diagnosis is that if it walks like a duck and quacks like a duck, it's probably a duck. This patient walked like a duck, and quacked like a duck, but turned out to be something very different.

Fortunately, his mind came back after several weeks of proper treatment for DTs caused by rapid alcohol withdrawal and the stress of surgery. What did I learn from this patient? There are very few "sure things" in medicine. There is always ambiguity. Complications, related or unrelated, may follow a technically perfect procedure. A complete, accurate medical history is very important and critical to proper treatment of the presenting problem. The patient's psychosocial history may be the most important information to collect and understand. I learned to always get a detailed psychosocial and medical history from the spouse since the patient may be living in denial. As I had learned back in grade school, the question is sometimes more important than the answer. The wrong question will only provide bad information. For example, the question, "How many drinks do you have every day" is more precise and less value-laden than "Are you a heavy drinker?"

The First Heart Transplant in Wisconsin

Nineteen sixty-eight continued to be a very interesting year. On October 21, 1968, I was present for the first heart transplant in Wisconsin performed by Dr. Derwood Lepley, Jr., eleven months after Dr. Christiaan Barnard's history-making first transplant. Dr. Lepley was one of the pioneers in cardiac revascularization and possibly the best cardiac surgeon in the Midwest.

The recipient was Betty Anick. Because of her deteriorating heart condition, Ms. Anick had been spending 22 hours a day in bed. She would not have lived longer than several months without a heart transplant. The donor was Robert Beulow. Mr. Beulow had suffered a massive head injury. He was "brain dead," having no cerebral function and very little brain stem activity. A ventilator controlled respirations, as his brain no longer regulated breathing. His body was being maintained using extraordinary means. His family was deeply involved. In accordance with Mr. Beulow's beliefs regarding advanced directives, they signed the consent to terminate life support.

The hospital's administrative, legal and medical staff and its chaplain had thoroughly prepared for this historic procedure. Betty Anick's priest had provided her and her family with counseling. Milwaukee County District Attorney and the Coroner's offices were part of the planning process. The day of the procedure, the patients were in surgical suites across a hall from each other. Several transplant teams were involved. Dr. Lepley headed the Anick team.

The heart/lung machine and pump technicians stood by with Dr. Lepley. Several teams and a representative of the Milwaukee County Coroner's Office staffed the Beulow suite. The cardiac monitors from both suites were visible from the hall. The anesthesiologist began the procedure in Dr. Lepley's suite.

A heart/lung bypass machine supported Betty. As Dr. Lepley removed her heart, the cardiac monitor flat lined. The source of electrical activity was out of her chest. As this was happening, the anesthesiologist for Mr. Beulow's teams turned off his respirator. Several minutes passed as his cardiac monitor began to register irregular beats. His heart finally went into ventricular fibrillation. The Milwaukee County Coroner pronounced Mr. Below dead and left the room as the surgical teams began their organ harvests.

About this time one of the surgical nurses discovered that the ice slush in the large narrow mouth flask had partially fused. The ice slush would not pour into the pan used to transport the heart between surgical suites. I did not have any training or experience with heart surgery, but being a good old boy from the south side of Milwaukee, I knew how to chop ice. I asked a scrub nurse for one glove and a Kocher (a long heavy straight hemostat clamp with teeth on the end). The nurse held the flask containing the fused ice on a table, and I chopped the ice through the narrow neck. She shook the ice out of the flask into the pan containing saline just as the team removed Mr. Beulow's heart.

His monitor changed from fibrillation to flat line. The other teams immediately went to work harvesting other organs (corneas, kidneys, liver) for other patients needing transplants. The heart was carried across the hall in the pan. When Dr. Lepley placed the heart into Betty's chest, her monitor changed from flat line to fibrillation. Dr. Lepley connected the plumbing—veins and arteries. A small open chest defibrillation paddle was placed on each side of the transplanted heart. Dr. Lepley shouted, "Clear!" and hit the switch. Betty's monitor changed from fibrillation to a normal rhythm as the transplanted heart began beating. The heart-lung bypass machine was removed and the chest closed. Betty lived a very active life for almost nine years following the transplant. Betty died of a heart attack at age 57 in 1977.

At the time, heart transplant was an experimental procedure and excluded from coverage by any insurance plan. St. Luke's Hospital absorbed the cost, and I am sure all the physicians worked *pro bono publico,* that is, without charging a fee. The procedure was as much about the publicity gained by St. Luke's demonstrating technological superiority as it was a humanitarian gesture toward Betty Anick. Whatever it was, it worked out well for all involved.

This spectacular achievement of medical technology occurred over forty years ago. The next year man was to walk on the moon. I voted for Richard Nixon in November of 1968. Hubert Humphrey never had a chance and the election was a landslide rejection of the Democrats and the Vietnam War. The war began to wind down. Detente was in and my draft number was never called. Since then medical technology has advanced, become more complex and more costly at an ever-increasing rate. In 1968, the cost of health care was well under 10 percent of our GNP. The cost of medicine today is approaching 18 percent, making American business and industry non-competitive in the world market.

In the middle of my rotating internship on December 22, 1968, our son Mark was born. If you are doing the math, both kids were born in the same year. Some people call that having "Irish Twins." Admitted early for observation with false labor, Kathy went into labor for real within forty-eight hours, just in time for an ice storm. Our obstetrician was not able to get to the hospital because of the ice, but I was the intern on call for that day. I had planned my internship obstetrics rotation for Kathy's expected date of confinement. I delivered my son, who weighed in at just less than six pounds.

A Crib Death—Almost

I had a very heavy schedule during the following several months working all days and twenty nights each month. Fortunately, our son, Mark, chose one of the mornings I was at home to stop breathing. My wife had gotten up early to nurse him when he went limp, stopped breathing and turned gray. She handed him to me as I sat on the edge of the bed. I did not know why he had stopped breathing. As I held him in my hands, I watched his neck for a few seconds, looking for a pulse. He still had a strong pulse so no cardiac compression would be needed. For a few seconds that seemed like an eternity I gave him small low pressure mouth-to-mouth puffs of air. He responded and opened his eyes.

My wife had dressed quickly and called the neighbor to sit with our one-year-old daughter. I called St. Luke's to let them know my son had been revived from a respiratory arrest and to have the emergency room ready. I was relieved to learn that our pediatrician, one of the best in Milwaukee, was on duty in the ER. He would be waiting for us. The old car started and we raced to St. Luke's Hospital.

Our son stopped breathing again at 6th Street and Oklahoma Avenue. I resuscitated him once more. St. Luke's Hospital is at 28th Street and Oklahoma. My wife must have made the last twenty-two blocks in less than two minutes, but it seemed a lot longer. Dr Kowalski met us at the emergency entrance, and quickly transported our son to the exam area. By this time he was pink, bright eyed, and for all appearances, a healthy two-month-old.

The nurse anesthetist mobilized for the emergency gave me one of those "harrumph" looks and asked with a patronizing tone, "Code Four, Dr. Strube?" Code Four was the short term used to describe a cardio-pulmonary arrest. Dr. Kowalski listened to Mark's chest and thought he heard sibilant rhonchi (squeaks) in the right lower lobe of the lungs. A chest x-ray showed only a questionable shadow in this area. Dr. Kowalski knew I was not an alarmist and, in spite of minimal objective findings, something very serious could be going on. He decided to admit my son for observation.

Kathy accompanied Mark to the pediatric unit on the fifth floor of the old building, and I walked to the cafeteria on the far end of the new building. I had been on a very serious diet and at this point knew I needed food just to stay on my feet. Just as they delivered my toast and coffee the voice over the hospital announced, "Code Four, Pediatrics, Room 512!" As I rounded the corner onto the long straight hall that connected the buildings, I saw Dr. Kowalski with the nurses and crash cart entering the elevators some 100 yards away. I reached the stairs near these elevators and flew up to the fifth floor. When I entered the room, Dr. Kowalski was inserting an endotracheal tube into Mark's windpipe and the nurse anesthetist was attempting to start an IV.

As Dr. Kowalski placed the tracheotomy tube, Mark went through a "Moro Reflex," indicating he was neurologically intact. My blood sugar must have bottomed out, as I sat on a wastebasket near the door. One of the nurses asked me if I wanted to see a Chaplain. I answered, "Call him if the son-of-a-bitch can start an IV."

Mark spent twenty-four hours on the pediatric Bird Respirator and several additional days in the hospital. He suffered no neurological damage. A cause for his respiratory arrest was never determined. I believe he would not be with us now if I had not been home that frigid February morning.

This dramatic episode taught me several things. The first is that medical personnel need to listen to their patients (and their families). The second, and probably most important for my later career, is that medical situations are not always clear and at times, the ambiguity may be crushing. Physicians practicing in the trenches must be given the benefit of the doubt from their patients, other physicians, managed care medical reviewers, insurance companies and politicians.

There were many times during my career as a managed care medical director when the documented history and physical findings of the patient did not completely match the standards and criteria for the requested procedure. That feeling I had at home with my son in my hands would come back. I would be in the trenches of front line family practice for the next fifteen years. I would frequently experience that feeling of uncertainty and frustration because of the ambiguity of the patient's problems.

Internship—The Second Half

I rotated through several medical and surgical services at St. Luke's during my year of internship. The interns were also assigned clinic duties. The hospital sponsored a "free clinic" where low income, underemployed, unemployed people and children were seen at no charge. The educational programs' director also managed the free clinics and had oversight for interns' scheduling, patient load and prescribing. This was a very low-pressure but satisfying part of the program because I felt we were helping people in need.

I "scrubbed in" and assisted in surgery with several very good orthopedic surgeons. I spent some time with the professionals in the Radiology Department, reviewing my clinic patients' X-ray films, and was very impressed with this group of professionals. The technology in the department was state-of-the-art.

Near the end of this year of internship, I passed Part Three of the National

Boards. The State of Wisconsin has reciprocity with the National Boards, so the State Board of Medical Examiners issued my License to Practice Medicine. I also obtained a federal license to prescribe controlled substances from the Federal Drug Enforcement Administration (DEA). I could now be considered a "general practitioner" and could have joined a medical group practice or started my own office.

My wife and I had two small children and I wanted to get on with life. I was eager to start making my mark practicing medicine. However, I understood the times were changing and the day of the "general practitioner" was coming to an end. To be successful in the long term, a physician needed to be certified by one of the American Medical Association boards of medicine or surgery.

As I have said, I enjoyed both orthopedic surgery and radiology very much. An orthopedic residency would mean another five years of training with a very stressful schedule of night call and emergency room coverage. It could mean a long commute or moving away from the grandparents to another city. The radiology residency would be three years with virtually no night call so, if necessary, some evenings could be devoted to reading the literature. The radiology residency was my logical choice.

Radiology Residency: 1969–1971

Starting in July 1969, I was accepted to start a three-year residency in Radiology at St. Luke's Hospital. I spent my first year of residency in diagnostic radiology. I also arranged to cover several evening shifts per month working for the physician group that held the contract to staff the St. Luke's Hospital Emergency Room. During the next several years, I worked the odd evening or weekend shift in the Trinity Hospital Emergency Room. This work kept my diagnostic and minor surgical skills sharp, and I enjoyed the direct patient contact.

Radiology is about visualizing three-dimensional anatomical structures using two-dimensional images to determine if an abnormality is present. A radiologist must have a very sound knowledge of anatomy and must be a highly skilled diagnostician. Although technology has changed dramatically and rapidly over a relatively short time, the professional and interpersonal dynamics among the patient, the attending physician and the radiologist remains the same.

Most procedures are simple routine imaging for uncomplicated problems. The attending physician orders the X-ray thought to be the most appropriate to establish the patient's diagnosis. The patient registers and is taken to the room where the diagnostic procedure is completed. In the old days, if the problem was serious, the radiologist with the resident at his side, read the X-ray film immediately after it emerged from the automatic processor. The radiologist called the physician with the result, and dictated a report.

The older docs called this a "wet reading," harkening back to the days when the film was hand dipped into developing tubs and a quick wet read did involve holding a dripping film in front of a view box. Very elderly physicians might order a "flat plate" of the abdomen. This terminology was from back in the days when X-ray departments produced images in a photographic emulsion on a glass plate.

The films from routine, non-urgent studies were loaded into a large view box that worked like the carpet rack at your local Home Depot. At the push of a button, the machine would rumble and another row of films would roll up into view. The films were read and reports dictated. The dictation was recorded on analog magnetic tape. For more complicated problems, the patients would be examined by the radiologist. A focused history and physical provide the radiologist with more information about the patient's condition. This additional information increases the likelihood of a high quality, accurate reading and report.

Many times the radiologist determined the attending physician had ordered an imaging study that would not be helpful, or that a more appropriate study could be done. The radiologist would call the attending physician to discuss the patient's problems and that a more appropriate study might provide better information.

During my training, the radiology department produced medical documents on paper. Computers were used for scheduling appointments and billing. Hospitals have become more sophisticated, but many community-based medical practices continue this model of paper charts and computerized appointment schedules and billing. Not much has changed for community medical practice in forty years.

The days of flat plates, wet readings and film are at an end. With the refinement of first analog and then digital high-definition imaging equipment, many radiologists now spend the majority of their days sitting in front of a computer screen. Reports dictated into a microphone connected to a computer using voice recognition software become a digital file. The electronic reports become computer files saved to the imaging category of the patient's medical record.

This information may remain electronic and instantly accessible within the hospital walls, but should not be confused with a "database" or "Problem-Oriented Electronic Medical Record" (POEMR). The computerized system is simply an electronic reproduction of a paper-based system, but with the ability to retrieve reports and consults much faster. Unfortunately, all this technology is typically then used to generate a report printed on paper and mailed to the attending physician. After review by the physician, a front office clerk places the paper report in a paper chart and buries it with other manila folders in a file cabinet.

The institutional billing for the procedure is electronic and directly communicated to the claim payer (e.g., insurance company, HMO, Medicare, or Medicaid). The claim information transmitted consists of a diagnostic code, billing code and dollar amount. If a payer questions the medical necessity of the procedure after receiving the electronic claim form, a paper report is printed and submitted with the appeal.

At the time of my residency, the physician was King and Blue Cross was Chancellor of the Exchequer. Very few people questioned the decisions of the King. Claims adjudicators limited denials to submissions that violated the terms and limitations of the insurance policy. As Mel Brooks said in his movie *History of the World, Part I,* "It's good to be the King."

I spent about a year and a half studying diagnostic radiology at St. Luke's Hospital where I had to assimilate a great deal of declarative knowledge and master a few procedures. The practicing radiologist has a broad knowledge of the physics of gamma radiation—how the machines produce gamma rays, how these rays are modified by the body and how the images are produced. The technology used to generate the radiation and visualize the images has advanced rapidly, but the basic science remains the same.

Understanding and working with the science and evolving with the technology provide the knowledge foundation for the radiologist, but the ability to visualize patterns and think in three dimensions is critical. In the residency program, the apprentice sits at the side of the mentor and learns to recognize patterns. Gradually most people refine their natural ability to recognize patterns present in imaging studies that, combined with some history and physical findings, allow them to diagnose a patient's problems accurately.

In this respect, training in radiology is not unlike training in other medical and surgical specialties. Residents observe attending physicians as they combine their memory of basic science and declarative medical knowledge with the patient's "pattern" of history and physical findings. Using global subjective judgment, a working diagnosis is made. The basic premise is: "If the bird walks like a duck, and quacks like a duck, it must be a duck." This system works much of the time because the bird *probably* is a duck. However, what happens if the bird turns out to be a swan or a goose? Memory-based global subjective judgment and probabilistic thinking applied to pattern recognition can frequently be a recipe for disaster. During flu season, a patient with headache, high fever and muscle aches will *probably* be diagnosed as having "the flu." There is a reasonable probability that the medical professional has arrived at the correct diagnosis. The patient is prescribed medications for symptomatic relief. However, if the patient has spinal meningitis, which has similar symptoms, death could be 24 hours away.

The radiology resident spends a great deal of training time viewing radiographic imaging studies while sitting beside the mentoring radiologist. Pattern recognition comes with practice to those residents with the basic capability. Dictating a concise accurate understandable report is a function of art, style, political awareness and mastery of grammar. Over time, the resident develops skill at reading imaging studies and dictating artful reports.

As a resident, I learned to "drive" the fluoroscope while performing barium enemas. These studies were diagnostic for some patients. Beyond diagnosing the cause of rectal bleeding or an abdominal mass, the procedure may be used therapeutically to resolve a bowel obstruction in an adult or to reduce an intussusception (the bowel telescoping inside itself) in a child. The X-ray technician shoots standard large format film images. The radiology resident usually dressed in surgical scrubs, wearing a lead apron, then drives the fluoroscope. The fluoroscope is used to visualize and shoot standard spot images.

A complete physical examination by any competent attending physician involves the use of at least one glove. Radiologists have been using lead shielded gloves since Madame Curie lost her fingers. The radiologist or resident uses gloved hand to move the barium contrast around in the colon and flatten out areas of the colon for better visualization. The free hand drives the fluoroscope and records pertinent still images.

If any area looked abnormal (pattern recognition again), additional images were recorded. These procedures involved close personal contact between the radiology resident and an apprehensive, physically uncomfortable patient lying on a cold hard X-ray table in a darkened alien environment undergoing a procedure to diagnose or resolve a serious, possibly life-threatening medical condition. Something was wrong with these patients, or they would not be on the table.

In those days, "preventive health" was an ill-defined abstraction and "screening" was something physicians ordered or did while chasing wild geese. Medical insurance evolved as a funding mechanism for the diagnosis and treatment of disease. The attending physician sometimes created references to signs and symptoms in the patient's chart to justify a preventive health-screening test or any unnecessary medical testing. The U.S. Public Health Service (later to become the U.S. Department of Health and Human Services) would not convene the Preventive Services Task Force until 1984, and no scientific universally acceptable standards for "prevention" or "screening" or "wellness" had yet developed.

These were the days when most tumors, including colon cancer, were discovered late. Most rectal cancers are within reach of the physician's index finger. If the patient reported blood in the toilet, a digital rectal exam was performed and a stool sample for blood was sent to the laboratory. Proctosigmoidoscopy to visualize the first eighteen inches of the colon, and a barium enema X-ray study would be done.

One of the most difficult procedural knowledge skills to master was the lymphangiogram (a study of the lymph nodes and system). This procedure used iodine-based radio opaque contrast dyes to highlight the lymph nodes along the spine in the abdomen and chest. Methyl blue dye was injected between the toes. This was picked up in the lymph channels, which could be seen under the skin. An extremely small butterfly needle was then inserted through the skin and into the lymph channel, now visible with the methyl blue dye. The radio opaque iodine-based contrast dye was injected using an electric motor-driven infusion pump. The iodine contrast would travel up the lymph channels and be filtered by the lymph nodes. X-rays were then taken of the pelvis, abdomen and chest to determine the character and size of the lymph nodes. The radiologist and resident would evaluate the films and dictate their findings, which were recorded and sent to transcription.

During my residency days, the viewing and dictating area was close to the secretaries' desks. This was in the day of the IBM Selectric Typewriters and White Out. One of the "girls" was our best typist. However, she was functioning with a couple of minor handicaps. Mary was a young, attractive, pleasant blonde, with rather large breasts and poor eyesight. The irregular staccato sound of her typing was constantly in the background as films were being read and reports dictated. Several times a day Mary's Selectric produced a regular drumming. Because of her poor eyesight, she would lean forward to check the report for errors and her breasts would press the space bar. Until word processors and laser printers replaced IBM Selectric typewriters, every time I heard the sound of a machine running off multiple spaces I had to smile.

Mary, or one of the other department administrative assistants, would type the report on a three-part NCR form. One copy for the therapy unit files, one for the hospital chart, and one for the attending physician's hospital mailbox. To this day, X-ray departments provide no copy of any diagnostic study to the patient without a written request. After the files resided on site for a specified period, the administrative staff boxed and moved the paper files to secure offsite storage.

The mailboxes near the doctor's entrance and lounge were for practicing physicians with hospital admission privileges. The physician would pick up the reports placed in these boxes and carry them to his office. Periodically, the staff administrative assistant would mail neglected reports to the ordering physician's office.

The physician office staff would (theoretically) notify the patient of the results and schedule the next visit. The paper reports would then be attached to the paper charts in the lab or X-ray findings section. All this paper would be buried in hospital and physician file cabinets in manila folders.

Radiation Therapy Training

St. Luke's Hospital had a highly-regarded and well-known radiation therapy unit where I spent six months studying the literature regarding the diseases treated using these machines. Not surprisingly, the vast majority of the patients treated in a radiation therapy unit have cancer and many have terminal diseases. Therapy procedures, whether invasive or non-invasive, do not have the pace of an active office practice; there is enough time to sit and talk with the patient and family. Sometimes cure is a possibility, and many discussions were about "cure rates" and probable limits on longevity. On a rare occasion, if questioned by the patient, the discussion would include the appropriateness of considering Hospice. These discussions were approached very carefully since most attending physicians did not want to be perceived as or could not emotionally tolerate "giving up" on trying to save their patients. Most attending physicians referred their patients to Hospice within days or weeks of the patient's death.

The radiation therapy unit was essentially a hospital-based consultation center. Patients evaluated there would have a complete history and physical and all the elements of a paper chart. The radiologist/radiotherapist is a medical doctor with training in radiology and usually advanced training through a fellowship in radiotherapy. Our chief of radiotherapy was one of the kindest, most thoughtful men I had ever met. The staff and the patients loved him. He had the respect and admiration of all the physicians on the hospital staff. I loved working with him, the staff and the patients.

The problem was that the practice of this specialty, by necessity, takes place in a basement bunker with walls and a ceiling several feet thick. The radiation had to be contained. The same basement area housed two very large hyperbaric chambers, initially built and installed for the heart surgery program, before development of the heart-lung machine. They were each the size of a small operating room. Picture a SCUBA tank ten feet in diameter and twenty-five feet long, with a massive air lock door at one end. The potential of a chamber exploding dictated the location. I had spent a little time on the hyperbaric service during my internship. These were the two quietest areas in the hospital.

The potential danger of these areas did not bother me, and interacting with and treating the patients was very satisfying on an emotional level. However, several months before the end of my second year, I realized life was too short to be spent in the shadows, both literally and metaphorically. Although a radiology practice is financially very lucrative, and the technology is fascinating and interaction with the patients can be rewarding, the work is typically done either in a basement bunker or in the core of a massive building. The location and lack of natural light was extremely oppressive. During winter, I would arrive at the hospital in the dark and leave in the dark after the last patient was treated. At least six months of the year the sun is not seen because of the short daylight hours and long working shifts. I did not have Seasonal Affective Disorder (SAD), but I realized a lifetime of this work would take its toll. I could end up a very grumpy old man. The most troubling issue for me, however, was the metaphoric shadows.

I had observed that many studies ordered by staff attending physicians were not medically necessary or that a more appropriate imaging study could be done. The radiologist could suggest a more appropriate X-ray or a special view that would be more helpful. The attending physician usually ordered the suggested test. Although most of the hospital attending staff appreciated the radiologists, some made it clear that they considered the professionals in that department as merely part of the machinery. They preferred that we simply view the ordered X-rays and dictate a report. The dictated reports had to be obfuscated to disguise this issue and not call the staff physician out. At the same time, the report had to justify the study so the hospital and radiologist would be paid their fees. This apparent truth was never stated, but it was abundantly clear that this was and would be the reality.

People have greater or lesser abilities to recognize patterns. Physicians who gravitate to radiology usually have very good pattern recognition abilities and enjoy discovering significant shapes in the random chaos of the images. X-ray images are patterns frozen in time on film or in digital files. Radiologists have to be very good at pattern recognition. Then they provide expert opinions about the patterns of the shadows they review.

Radiologists generally provide high-quality, error-free reports. However, quality is not defined as what the credentialed, certified medical expert reports or does. This applies not only to radiology, but also to all medical testing, imaging, procedures and treatments. The question regarding the quality of reporting produced by a radiology department is more about the medical necessity of the imaging ordered by the staff physicians than it is about the accuracy of the reports produced by the radiologists.

The evaluation of the quality of any radiology service requires answers to critically important questions. Key questions include:

- Is the radiologist a consultant to the patient, or a technician doing the biding of a staff physician, no matter how ludicrous the demand? The the function of the radiologist is the central question.
- How many of the studies or procedures were not medically necessary?
- How many studies were not relevant to the patient's problems?
- Did physicians order studies for one problem that prevented proper evaluation of another, possibly more serious problem?
- How many studies were done even though physicians knew no change would be made in the patient treatment plan?

Studies published in the Dartmouth Atlas[2] confirm my observation that a high percentage of imaging studies and other tests and procedures are not medically necessary and often inappropriate. In fact, the amount of money spent on medical problems does not necessarily mean that physicians are delivering better care. As a Dartmouth Atlas Briefing Paper states, "Atlas research shows that spending is inversely correlated with the likelihood of receiving recommended care."[3] These issues were becoming readily apparent as I made my way through my chosen career.

I realized my career choice expectations did not coincide with the practical world of a radiology practice. When I chose to enter the training program, my initial perception of what the residency and practice of radiology would be was a fantasy. During the next two years, the reality of life as a practicing radiologist became evident. Some physicians are well suited to this life. I was not.

I discussed my feelings with the head of the department and the head of the residency program. I stayed on to the end of my second year and during the last several months arranged to join a group practice that had been in Cudahy, Wisconsin, for many years. I would be "coming home" to my original dream of practicing medicine on the south side of Milwaukee.

---

2   See, for example, <u>Regional and Racial Variation in Primary Care and the Quality of Care Among Medicare Beneficiaries</u> (retrieved on January 18, 2011 from http://www.dartmouthatlas.org/downloads/reports/Primary_care_report_090910.pdf) and "Supply-Sensitive Care." A Dartmouth Atlas Project Topic Brief (retrieved on January 18, 2011 from http://www.dartmouthatlas.org/downloads/reports/supply_sensitive.pdf)

3   "Effective Care." A Dartmouth Atlas Project Topic Brief. Page 2. Retrieved on January 18, 2011 from http://www.dartmouthatlas.org/downloads/reports/effective_care.pdf.

PART TWO
Private Medical Practice
1971–1985

CHAPTER 3:
Medical Practice

I joined Fine-Lando Clinic during the summer of 1971 following the completion of two years of the three-year residency at St. Luke's Hospital. Dr. Fine and Dr. Lando had treated members of my family at various times over the years. The clinic they started had originally been in Dr. Fine's large home. Over time, as the clinic grew and physicians were added to the practice, the home was expanded. The practice finally outgrew the facility and new offices were built several blocks from Trinity Hospital. This facility was only a few years old when I joined.

Two Jewish physicians started the clinic. They had judiciously added physicians with various board specialty certifications as the need became evident. All the doctors were competent. The clinic was like a mini United Nations. There were Indian and Egyptian internists. One of the surgeons was Pakistani and the other was "Persian" from Iran. The cardiologist was German. The clinic had lab and X-ray facilities available on site. For more complex studies, the patient would be sent to Trinity Hospital.

The hospital staff showed even more diversity. My wife's obstetrician was born in Italy but trained in America. My favorite orthopedic surgeon was Irish. Referrals were made to the Japanese neurosurgeon. The neurologist was Canadian. Several Internists were from the Philippines. The American-born and foreign-born graduates of American medical schools appeared, at least on the surface, to function as one big happy family. We were all Americans. For many years as I practiced family medicine, I was not aware of any primal tribal rivalries. Nevertheless, pride, prejudice and politics would eventually surface.

Group Practice: 1971 to 1973

The clinic's physicians were all employees of the corporation but internally organized into informal partnerships of the two physicians. Each physician, by specialty, had an assigned alternate. These partners covered each other on alternate weekends and during vacations. Prior to starting practice, I was designated Dr. Lando's alternate. Shortly after I started work, I was reassigned to one of the other general practitioners. I believe a major disagreement developed between two of the younger physicians who served as each other's alternate. As a result, Dr. P became Dr. Lando's alternate. I became the alternate for Dr. C.

Six months after joining the clinic during the winter of 1971, we purchased a home in South Milwaukee near Trinity Hospital. We hosted a large gathering of friends and family at our new home at Christmas. Life was good for the first year. I continued working the occasional odd shift in the Trinity Emergency Room. My practice at the clinic continued to grow rapidly.

Private practice within the clinic was a real joy. The clinic's nurses were friendly, competent people who were very helpful as I learned the ropes of clinic practice. Hospital admitting privileges were virtually instantaneous because Fine-Lando Clinic was the most powerful group on Trinity's staff. Most of the hospital staff committee chairs were clinic physicians. After scrubbing with credentialed specialists several times, the surgeons made recommendations to approve additional privileges.

My privileges soon included normal vaginal deliveries, circumcision, dilatation and curettage (D&C), cervical conization, and tonsillectomy and adenoidectomy (T&A). I could perform a T&A in about nine minutes, including the wait for the bleeding to stop. The procedure was reasonably simple when performed on preadolescent children with huge tonsils. After the patient was anesthetized, the nurse anesthetist inserted the endotracheal tube. I then incised the anterior tonsillar pillars from near the base of the tongue, up to the soft palette using a hook-shaped scalpel. Using a Kocher clamp, I grasped the tonsil through the incision, then retracted and teased it away from surrounding tissues using a small, blunt, curved instrument.

Dr. Lando told me that in the old days (he was in his 70s at the time) many surgeons grew a long fifth fingernail for use in dissecting the tonsil away from the base. The human mouth, after all, is not a sterile place. The clamp on the tonsil was released and a wire snare was slid over the tip of the clamp. The tonsil was grasped once again and retracted as the snare was slid down the clamp and around the tonsil down to its base. Squeezing the handle a few times ratcheted the wire loop into the barrel of the snare, clipping the tonsil off.

Following the removal of the other tonsil, an adenotome was used to remove the adenoids. The adenotome is a long instrument similar to the snare but with a curved stainless steel box at the business end. The outside of the curve has a guillotine-like blade that closes like a roll top desk when the handle is squeezed. The small guillotine box is positioned up behind the soft palate, pushed into the adenoidal tissue and the handle is squeezed. The adenoids are clipped out.

The hardest part of the procedure was the wait for the bleeding to stop and resisting the temptation to do something about it. I would wrap my gloved hands in a sterile towel, sit on a stool and watch the clock for five minutes. Dr. Lando taught me to wait five minutes before looking for trouble, so I would not get carried away suturing or cauterizing blood vessels. In a healthy individual, these clean cut vessels would usually retract, constrict down and stop bleeding within three minutes. The wait was not to avoid the difficult process of tying off catgut sutures in the back of the throat, but rather to avoid the predictable bleed that occurs in the middle of the night a week later when the suture or cauterized tissue falls off.

Adults, because of chronic scar tissue that holds blood vessels open, tend to bleed more than kids do. After several years of doing tonsillectomies, I had placed only one suture, and that was in an adult. There is also a traditional belief among surgeons that red-haired patients are bleeders. I had not seen any scientific basis for this belief, and the concept may have been one of those unfounded assumptions passed on for centuries. However, I always waited five minutes before checking for bleeding for any red-haired patient.

Back then, tonsillectomy had two indications for proceeding. One was the presence of tonsils, and the other was Blue Cross coverage. Of course, documenting large tonsils and a history of several bouts of tonsillitis were helpful in justifying the procedure. However, the doctor did not need Blue Cross to approve it in order to schedule and perform the procedure. Back then, the doctor was king and it was good to be king. Blue Cross would pay for a tonsillectomy regardless of its justification; unnecessary procedures were not uncommonly used as a preventative measure.

Doing the "Thing Right" and Doing the "Right Thing"

I added this description to show that tonsillectomy, like many other surgical procedures, is neither complex nor time-consuming. I started doing this procedure when I was twenty-nine years old after four years at the university, four years of medical school, a year of internship and two years of residency. I assisted during many minor surgeries like this, most of which were equally simple. I believe I was very good at performing these surgical procedures, but I also believe a sixteen-year-old with excellent hand-eye coordination, skill with tools and the ability to tolerate the sight of blood could be taught to do the procedure in a very short time.

The sixteen-year-old, however technically competent, might not have the wisdom to understand appropriate treatment. Procedural skill is important, but determining if the procedure should be done is more important. It is important to do the *thing right* (technical skill) but may be more important to do the *right thing* (medical judgment). If a technically perfect tonsillectomy is performed resulting in an excellent outcome, but the procedure was not medically necessary, can it be said that quality medical care was delivered? During the 1970s, the concept of quality was poorly understood. To this day, it remains so for most physicians. Back then, standards of care and quality criteria were virtually non-existent. The standard of care was the "community standard," meaning just about anything the doctor ordered.

Since the 1980s, physician specialty societies, the AMA and many private medical research organizations have developed criteria and standards for many procedures and treatments. Some of these groups develop science-based standards—others, not so much. No longer do small groups of credentialed good old boys, sitting around a table using their unassisted memory to swap war stories and personal opinions, develop these standards of care.

Standards and criteria are now based on conclusions derived from statistically significant clinical epidemiological studies published in the peer reviewed medical literature. Insurance company bean counters do not formulate medical criteria to deny medically necessary care to policyholders. Peer reviewed scientific studies are evaluated and standards determined by panels of physicians trained in the science of clinical epidemiology and statistics. In spite of wide distribution of these written criteria and standards of care by many professional organizations, physicians continue to fall short of compliance with these standards and well short of delivering quality care.

My patient load grew rapidly so that by the end of my first year I was one of the clinic's top producers, as measured by patient visits, pharmacy billing and lab/X-ray studies ordered. Looking back, I am sure this rapid growth was not the result of the quality of care I delivered to my patients, since this did not significantly differ from my colleagues. My advantage may have been my middle class background and ability to relate to and communicate with patients.

My work in the emergency room was generating new patients for other clinic physicians as well as myself. The "production results" presented by the clinic administrator to the medical staff at the monthly business meetings were interesting, and I believed my financial results were not influencing my medical decision-making. I was seeing many patients, treating them to the best of my ability and believed they were receiving quality medical care.

However, at that time I knew nothing about quality. Given my education and training, how could I know? I know the tonsillectomies I preformed were technically sound and I would like to believe they were all medically necessary, but looking back, I cannot be sure. I was learning good technical skills and habits from my mentors, but did I learn the most up-to-date standards of care derived from scientifically based clinical epidemiology? Was I selecting patients for the procedure based on questionable traditions passed down in the clinic? Were financial incentives influencing the care I delivered? I believed at the time I was performing a necessary service, but looking back knowing what I know now, I cannot deny that I may have been influenced by some subjective or arbitrary consideration. Lacking standards of care and an appropriate "checklist," it is impossible to say that I performed these procedures to the standards of care I am now advocating.

Virtually all the clinic's patients or their dependents were working people, and all had some form of medical insurance. The insurance industry as a sector of the economy or as a concern of big business was not newsworthy. The economics of medical care delivery or the financial reality of operating a medium-sized clinic was not a conscious concern of mine, or of many other medical staff folks. I believed my patients were receiving the best care available for their problems, but the cost of that care was not my issue. By seeing thirty clinic patients per day, having twenty admissions per month, performing ten minor surgical procedures per month and delivering fifty babies per year, I made a very good living.

The economic impact of health care on American business was no one's concern. I was working hard, loving what I was doing and financially very comfortable. Doctors like me could suppress the financial realities and imagine our concern was strictly about the optimal well-being of our patients. Spending other people's money provides that kind of satisfaction, and we were happy thinking we were providing the best care possible regardless of cost.

The In-Patient "Banker's Physical" Evaluation

At that time, the benefit structure of Blue Cross and most other insurance companies was based on covering the medical expenses generated by the hospital-based treatment of catastrophic medical conditions. They paid reasonably well for the bills generated when the physician treated any patient in the hospital. Insurance companies established exclusions, co-payments, deductibles and lifetime maximums to control costs by shifting payment responsibility to the patient. The physician was not required to justify the medical necessity for anyone's admission.

Indemnity insurance plans offered no coverage for many outpatient medical services. Some outpatient services, such as preventive health care, were severely restricted or not covered. The industry believed these services were inexpensive and easily paid out of pocket by the patient—classic economists would say they were externalizing costs to the individual, not understanding that the psychology of self-care includes too much denial and procrastination for this formula to work well. Instead of focusing on preventative care, the industry chose to attempt to reduce utilization and slow the relentless increase in costs through benefit package redesign and other financial manipulations. These attempts have failed.

Even if the physician was still king (and it was still good), they did have to periodically fight insurance companies to pay the bills. Insurance executives of all stripes forget that physicians were some of the most intelligent students in school—and must be to be able to get through the medical school vetting process. Why would physicians, after graduating from medical school and completing a residency, suddenly develop a terminal case of stupidity? To mitigate outpatient reimbursement problems, doctors admitted many patients to the hospital for testing.

The "Banker's Physical" that was in vogue provided patients the illusion of complete, executive service. Without evidence-based scientific standards of care, vast numbers of unnecessary admissions and tests were ordered. If a new patient was found to have hypertension and good insurance coverage, most physicians would admit the patient. They would evaluate kidney anatomy and function using a battery of stressful invasive tests.

Physicians admitted patients to the hospital for a couple of days. The hospital administration was happy to have the admissions and the billing for the technological component of the testing. The hospital-based radiologists and pathologists appreciated the business. The private clinic administration happily billed for the admitting physician's professional hospital visit component. The patient was satisfied with what they perceived as "high quality" health care. Blue Cross was happy with the profit (a.k.a., *retained earnings* in a not-for-profit entity) from processing the claims on a "cost plus" basis. At the time, the cost of health care, including all the unnecessary testing and procedures was not unreasonable. Unlike today, health care was not driving employers off shore or out of business—or forcing many patients into bankruptcy.

"Health" insurance is a misnomer and always has been. Blue Cross and all other companies, public and private, essentially provide "sickness" insurance. The concept of "wellness" had not caught on before the 1990s, and to most physicians, immunizations were the only form of prevention they recognized. The U.S. Preventive Services Task Force would not be convened until 1984 and would meet for five years before the first guidelines defining effective preventive health screening studies were published. Since 1989, the guidelines have been published by the Federal Government and are available to download free on the Health and Human Services website (http://www.hhs.gov/safety/index.html).

Until publication of these studies and guidelines began in 1989, no organization offered the mechanism to develop standards for "screening" and each physician ordering the test individually defined preventive health. The best qualification and one of the major incentives for a "complete inpatient work-up" for any problem was the presence of Blue Cross–Blue Shield insurance. Health care delivery was not based on scientific evidence. Both the physician and the patient believed they were spending other people's money, which made it easier to order unnecessary tests. For most patients and physicians, this remains the case.

Over the next thirty-seven years, medical consumption skyrocketed in spite of broad development of medical criteria and standards. Professional journals published this information and physician organizations provided wide distribution through direct mailings. Continuing medical education seminars provided physicians with information needed to describe standards of care. All attempts to improve health care quality by increasing the individual physician's knowledge base have failed. Utilization of medical services accelerated and overutilization became much worse. Gross overutilization is now termed "abuse."

Striving for Efficiency

During the 1970s, efficiency of care was my concern, but cost of care was rarely an issue. Still, growing up as I did in a lower middle class family where finances were always tight, I disliked spending other people's money foolishly, almost as much as I disliked spending my own. When I admitted patients to the hospital, I wanted a good medical reason to do so and would try to get them back home as soon as possible.

I learned early on that the patient's psychosocial situation was as important to understand as their medical condition. I could shorten hospital stays for my patients using the very simple technique of writing a "Social Service Consult for Discharge Planning" as part of the admission orders. The idea was to prepare for discharge on the day of admission. Other physicians accumulated many unnecessary hospital days because they did not put in place a thoughtful discharge plan early during the admission process.

The hospital's social workers had all the contacts to arrange home nursing, durable home medical equipment, and admission to a rehabilitation facility or nursing home. A hospice referral could be facilitated by such a referral. In the cases that wanted them, the hospital chaplains were also very comforting to the patient and family.

However, planning for discharge was not enough. A timely discharge order had to be written. Because I was making rounds twice a day, I could modify the treatment plan if necessary based on the condition of the patient and the results of the day's testing. Sometimes the discharge order could be written for the following day. Morning hospital rounds assessed the patient's condition, and tests that had not been posted on the chart the prior evening could be reviewed. If the patient was stable and discharge planning was complete, the discharge order was written. A morning discharge order meant the patient could go home before noon, eliminating an additional hospital day from the cost of the stay. An added benefit was that most stable patients recover better at home than through an unnecessarily extended hospital stay.

During the fall of 1972, Dr. Lando had scheduled a fishing vacation to the Florida Keys. At one of the monthly meetings, my alternate objected to his timing because it was during the clinic's busy season. I knew my alternate and the rest of the primary care physicians could cover his practice without a problem, since he had been slowing down in preparation for retirement. I voiced this opinion at the meeting, not understanding office politics and potential repercussions. The Board allowed Dr. Lando the time off for his fishing trip. Coverage for his patients during the busy flu season that winter went very smoothly, but this was not the end of the story.

The Beginning of the End

Just after the new year began in 1973, an internist with more seniority than me was up for partnership. He was from the Philippines. Partnership would have meant voting rights at the clinic meetings and progressive ownership of shares in the clinic facility. Although he was an excellent physician and qualified for partner status, the good old boys wanted no additional partners.

My impression was that the existing partners did not want to dilute the power or ownership structure any further. It was abundantly clear that the rest of the newcomers would not be offered a piece of the pie when the time came. This strategy ultimately led to the decline of the power of the clinic, both in the community and on the hospital staff.

Shortly after this situation unfolded, I scheduled a ten-day summer family vacation five months in advance and posted the dates on the clinic calendar. My wife and I selected the Fourth of July week so we could participate in the major South Shore Yacht Club sailing race to Grand Haven, Michigan. I thought this would be a good time to be away from the clinic since medical offices usually slow down during summer, especially since many families vacation in July and August. Business does not pick up again until it is time for children to return to school.

The clinic cancelled our scheduled vacation a month after the posting. My alternate felt it would be too much of a burden to cover my patients. My alternate was the same clinic physician that had opposed Dr. Lando's yearly bone fishing vacation. I felt the cancellation of my family vacation was payback for supporting the senior partner's vacation request the previous winter. No good deed goes unpunished.

During the winter following the cancellation of my summer family vacation, the clinic board made a request that I give up working in the emergency room so I could focus on clinic patients. Patients I treated at Trinity ER were billed through the clinic. The clinic took 10 percent for this billing service. Clinic board members reviewed the monthly financial reports. The addition of the ER billing to my clinic production made me one of the top producers. Perhaps some on the board felt I was too productive. It did not matter. I began to make plans to set up my own practice.

I consulted my lawyer and accountant regarding a proper exit strategy. My contract with the clinic was set to expire on July 1, 1973. It would need to be honored, but I wanted to give the clinic and patients proper notice of my intent to leave. I did not intend to give up working at the emergency room. There was a probability that the clinic would accept my resignation immediately upon notice, as is the usual custom and best business decision for the organization.

I had confidential discussions with local medical office personnel and had a complete small office staff prepared to submit a two-week notice of resignation to their employers. There were several available office spaces in the Cudahy and South Milwaukee area that, with some remodeling, would be suitable. My banker was a personal friend and had taken care of my family for years. I had the papers ready for a small business loan.

I submitted my written notice of resignation on April 1st to be effective July 1st, giving the clinic three months notice. The clinic held an emergency meeting and accepted my resignation immediately. Since they had terminated my employment early and without cause, they were obligated not to cancel the contract. As a result, the clinic continued to pay my monthly checks for the "tail" on my accounts receivable through the end of June. Since they had broken the contract, the non-compete clause was invalid. I had experienced group practice, and it was time to move on.

I knew my relationship with the physicians of the Fine-Lando Clinic was not over since I would be practicing in the area for years to come. The Academy Award winning, second best picture of all time, "The Godfather," was released in March 1972, just before I completed my first full year at the clinic. As I walked out of the clinic, carrying a box of personal items, I recalled an important concept from the movie. The action taken by the clinic was not personal. It was a sound business decision.

Solo Practice: 1973 to 1978

The three weeks following my last day at the Fine-Lando Clinic were hectic, although I had prepared well for the predictable outcome following my three-month notice of resignation. Kathy and I had privately discussed our possible need for a small business bridge loan with our banker, a friend at Cudahy Marine Bank where our home mortgage was held.

I had been talking to the owner of a small old red brick commercial building on the northwest corner of Packard and East Barnard Avenues in downtown Cudahy. This corner building was right out of a Norman Rockwell illustration. Frank's Drug Store was the small business on the first floor.

The second floor had originally been an apartment used as living quarters for the business owner when the building was constructed. The street entrance to the second floor was through a door at the side of the drugstore. Once inside, a long steep stairway led to the original apartment some fourteen feet above the street level. The climb would prove to have a significant "natural selection" impact on the cross section of patients I would see in this office. Serving a younger, more mobile population would have a positive effect on my professional and private life.

The original second floor living quarters consisted of a back stairwell, kitchen, and pantry, a dining room overlooking Barnard Avenue to the south, and a front room overlooking Packard Avenue to the east. The front stairwell, middle bedroom, bathroom and back bedroom were on the north half. The front stairwell wound around a small closet off the front living room. We immediately saw the promise in this location and the space. The front living room closet would become the record room; the pantry would become lab space and the back bedroom would become an X-ray facility.

Manfred Landsberg, M.D., had used this space several years earlier as a physician's office, so the community was used to having a small practice in the building and the rooms had already been converted for practical use as an office. He lived in Bay View within blocks of where I grew up. Coincidentally, back in high school, his daughter, Tina, had been part of our circle of friends. The offices were rather dark and dingy, since they had been not been occupied or redecorated in a very long time. All the office and medical equipment were gone. Dr. Landsberg had apparently used the back bedroom for his X-ray equipment. The bedroom closet had the plumbing in place for a film-developing tank. The black walls and chemical stains on the floor matched the mental picture from my medical school rotation through radiology at Milwaukee County General Hospital.

During the three weeks following my exit from the group practice, the entire workspace was redecorated and remodeled. Some work was subcontracted to repair people I knew, but friends and relatives volunteered most of the work. The grandmothers watched Jill and Mark, allowing Kathy and me to put in sixteen-hour days. Our fathers became part of the remodeling crew in the evenings since both were employed full-time.

A phone number was acquired and phones installed. Patients began calling almost immediately. Kathy answered the phone, scheduling appointments during the day when she was not painting moldings. At night, she sewed curtains and prepared patient charts. New vinyl tile and carpeting were laid on the floors. All the walls were painted or paneled. We installed a drop ceiling in several rooms, and other ceilings were painted.

I wired new fixtures in all rooms and installed a sound system. The pantry was converted into a lab and lab equipment was purchased. Used X-ray equipment was purchased and installed in the back exam room. A developing tank was installed in the closet off this room. Nearing the end of remodeling, each exam room was fitted with white metal overhead cabinets and sinks ordered from Sears weeks before. Several used examination tables were purchased and moved into exam rooms. All new exam room medical equipment was purchased and installed.

Patients had been calling for appointments during the remodeling and several dropped in to view the continuing progress. Many times, I would be working there with a hammer in my hand and wearing bib overalls when a patient stopped in to see the progress. None of our visitors believed the office would be ready for the opening day. Miraculously, three weeks after I left the group practice, the doors of my new, fully staffed, completely remodeled and equipped office opened.

Kathy became the administrator and bookkeeper with the assistance of our accountant. My nurse managed the professional staff. I saw twelve patients the first day. I had transitioned from being an employee of a medium-sized medical group with no administrative or financial concerns to being a solo medical practitioner with all the risks and responsibilities of a small business owner.

The effort of remodeling and organizing a physical location and the paperwork involved initiating a small business were not the only considerations. This was not just a small business. It was a medical practice and all the paperwork and notifications that accompany such a special purpose endeavor had to be completed before any of our efforts would bear fruit. Notifications of address change and business name had to be sent and acknowledged by the State Licensing Board, American Medical Association, State Medical Society, Milwaukee Medical Society, Federal DEA Office and Blue Cross Blue Shield (BCBS), the major indemnity insurer in the area. All these issues were managed for me when I was part of a clinic, but now I had to get my own ducks in a row.

As a "new" practitioner, BCBS had no billing profile for me. I needed to establish my charges for all the procedures I would perform. The codes for procedures are standardized, but, in theory, all physicians (or clinics) establish their own fees for each service listed. This had something to do with antitrust legislation and professionals not being allowed to get together to set fees. The idea was that if the providers were in competition, the consumer would be able to find quality service at the lowest price.

In reality, a standard BCBS schedule was readily available. Because of sunshine laws that have more recently become useful, Medicare and Medicaid publish their rates and, by law, require that no provider contract for a lower rate with any payer or purchaser. Back then, many practices had very similar fee-for-service (FFS) schedules based on the BCBS Resource Based Relative Value Scale. Some fees might differ slightly, but essentially they were all very close.

So how were adjustments for inflation made and how would a doctor know when the BCBS fee multiplier went up? BCBS would adjust their reasonable and customary fee schedule with inflation but when and how would this happen? Since I do not recall how this actually happened and have no memory of who was involved, the following parable may help explain how a mythical insurance company communicated fee schedule increases.

Fee-for-Service Fee Determination:
An Allegory and the Reality

Once upon a time, long ago in the far away mythical land where physicians delivered quality, low-cost care for all the people, rich and poor, young and old alike, a small group of unknown Medical Society minions determined the cost of the new Cadillac had gone up 5 percent. The physicians would therefore need a 5 percent cost-of-living raise. This secret society of negotiators met with an equally secret and anonymous group of negotiators from the insurance giant, *Seguros del Doble Cruz Azul* (SDCA), to determine the new fee multiplier.

The SDCA negotiators had determined that the cost of a new Lincoln had gone up only 4 percent. They insisted that a new Lincoln was equivalent to a new Cadillac. After a night of tough negotiation in a private room in the basement of one the finest German restaurants in the land, they would decide on 4.5 percent as the cost-of-living increase. SDCA then passed this increase cost on to the citizens.

In due course, an anonymous employee in every physician's office would get a call from an unknown person in the Medical Society, and would be told the new "multiplier" had increased to 1.045. The $100 service would become $104.50. All other services rendered by this physician would also go up by about 4.5 percent. Bookkeepers in this land had developed an easily administered, simple system that kept up with inflation, and no one went to jail for price fixing.

Determining fees in the mythical land was just that simple, and all physicians delivered quality, low-cost care. It worked well until, as the years rolled by, medical entrepreneurs introduced many expensive technologically advanced tests and procedures. The practice of medicine became more complex. Then the citizens discovered that not all physicians provided quality, low-cost care. Some physicians had determined they needed a Rolls Royce instead of a Lincoln and focused on improving their bottom line rather than their patient's health. The end of the system came as it failed to provide appropriate, effective, accessible, efficient health care. Soon HMOs came to the land to address the quality and cost problems—but that is a story for later.

The reality of fee determination in a fee-for-service system was not nearly so simple as the allegory above (which, at some level, many people believe). Kathy and I had worked our way through school and upon my graduation from Marquette Medical School, we had no student loans to pay off. However, the bridge loan from the Cudahy Marine Bank for the office remodeling and equipment was significant, and we had the mortgage and other expenses for the home we had purchased in South Milwaukee to cover. In addition to servicing the small business loan, there would be salaries to pay, Federal/State income tax to be withheld, monthly supplies to purchase, utilities to pay, malpractice insurance premiums, and health care insurance for my family and our employees. We had gone over the numbers with my accountant and understood I had to generate $70 per hour just to meet our business obligations before we could pay Kathy or me a salary. Every medical provider has to do his or her own calculations along these lines to determine their fee structure—everyone's bills are slightly different, so fees can differ significantly.

At the time, although I did not know the scope of utilization, quality and cost problems in the delivery system, I did understand that many physicians were providing excessive and unnecessary services. Lacking the education, training and experience in quality improvement, I did not know how to address these major issues, but I did understand that fee or wage controls would not work. In 1973 in our office, the fee for an uncomplicated office visit was under $10. Minor office surgery, lab and X-ray fees would supplement this. We never failed to pay the bills or payroll, but there were a few lean months for Kathy and me in the beginning. By the time January 1974 rolled around, we had a reliable, steady income and could institute a defined contribution retirement plan for all full-time employees.

The Solo Practice: Working Today, Planning for Tomorrow

In these early years of solo practice, I did not work under the expectation that Social Security would be there for me in later years. I understood that our government had put "old age assistance" in place to prevent the elderly from starving in the streets, not to provide a comfortable retirement for anyone (I have been pleasantly surprised that Kathy and I are actually receiving small monthly Social Security checks since we turned 65). Kathy and I established a defined contribution plan to pay for retirement with banking, accounting and legal professional help. We had a lot to learn about small business; however, the future looked bright and we were very optimistic.

My policy of writing "Social Service Consult for Discharge Planning" as part of my admission orders significantly shortened hospital stays. I developed a cooperative relationship with the Trinity Hospital Social Services Department and the social workers on the staff. Through these folks, I acquired extensive knowledge of compliance with Medicare and Medicaid requirements. They also helped me understand the workings of the post-hospitalization resources, including the availability of nursing home and rehabilitation center beds and services provided by durable medical equipment suppliers.

We actively worked with local hospice care providers. Several of my elderly patients had been transferred from Trinity to a nursing home in South Milwaukee. The nursing home needed a medical director. I applied for and secured the position. Such positions are not difficult to secure, since very few physicians are interested in treating patients in "heaven's waiting room." Practicing physicians would generally discharge their patients needing minor rehabilitation or custodial care from the hospital to a nursing home.

Most of the time, care of the patient while in the facility would be transferred to the nursing home medical director. The duties were not burdensome. I would receive an urgent call regarding a medical problem or a not-so-urgent call regarding the need for my signature on a death certificate every once in a while. Once a month, I made rounds on all assigned patients to assess status and renew medications.

I learned very quickly that most of the patients were over-medicated with costly brand-name drugs. All these elderly patients were private pay or welfare admissions. I considered it an ethical and moral absolute that these people receive quality care at the lowest possible cost. For patients and their families paying for nursing home fees out of their own pockets, preserving resources was a big priority. Additionally, appropriate, effective, and efficient utilization of resources was a financial necessity for the nursing home due to government constraints on Medicaid reimbursement.

Quality care is only meaningful relative to the patient's overall medical and psychosocial realities. Many of these folks had terminal conditions. They had signed living wills and advanced directives. These documents typically specified they did not want any artificial means of life support. They directed the medical staff not to attempt resuscitation should they suffer a cardiac arrest.

For a person with a terminal cancer, having three to six months to live, continuing high cost medications to reduce cholesterol and continuing the recommended regular blood testing are not only pointless, but inappropriate medical care. The pharmacist and I evaluated the medication list for each patient to determine if each drug was the most appropriate for the problems and conditions being treated and if an equivalent generic were available. After discussions with the patient and family, drug and other therapies were tailored to each patient's individual uniqueness, goals and psychosocial realities. Doing so was neither complex nor time-consuming and, in my view, the essence of quality care.

Congress passed the Health Maintenance Organization Act of 1973 (Public Law 93-222), also known as the HMO Act of 1973, 42 U.S.C. § 300e. President Nixon signed the act into law. I had no idea of the impact this initial legislation would have on the American health care system and paid little attention to the details of the bill or the politics involved. The prevailing opinion in the medical community was that HMOs were a bad idea. This new law was considered unworkable and the general public feeling was that it would have little impact on our lives. In fact, this initial HMO legislation had little impact for several years, but it turned out to be the proverbial "nose of the camel in the tent." This legislation would be revised and modified over time and by the 1990s would have a significant impact on medical cost and quality care issues.

Cudahy High School Team Physician

Soon after opening this practice, I met an old friend who was teaching history at Cudahy High School. We had been Milwaukee County lifeguards years before. Although Bernie had been a swimmer but never played football, he had been asked to join the Cudahy High School football coaching staff because of his enthusiasm and popularity as a history teacher.

Although initially he knew little about the game, he spent six months reading everything he could get his hands on regarding football strategy, tactics and coaching. For him, it was like studying the history of great military battles. His research and commitment paid off since his coaching staff took the Cudahy teams to the top of the suburban rankings for years.

The team physician was a local dermatologist who was not interested in continuing in the position. Bernie asked me to stop at the school to meet the other coaches. I became the Cudahy team physician that fall. Bernie has remained a good friend to this day.

Being on the Cudahy sidelines during the games was a joy, especially when South Milwaukee was the opponent. I also became a volunteer physician at the Bay View High School (a City of Milwaukee school) games, which I always attended. The Cudahy games were held Friday evenings and the Bay View games Saturday afternoons. All city games had been moved to daylight hours because of crowd control issues after dark.

In the suburban conference, the home team provided an ambulance on site and a game physician to manage any player injury. If an ambulance came to a Milwaukee game, it was because a fan had lost a fight and needed to be taken to the hospital. I attended all Cudahy home games and some of the away games. The coaches were all students of the game. They became experts at recognizing the offensive and defensive patterns of the other teams. The Cudahy football team was well prepared to execute counter measures to anything an opponent might throw at them.

The coaching staff attended the Booster Club meetings where the game films would be shown to the parents and hometown fans. After a win, these town hall gatherings were celebrations with kudos all around for the players. Of course, sometimes things would go badly in spite of excellent training, practice, preparation and coaching decisions. Outcomes were never predictable because of the variable and unique skill levels of the players and the bounce of the ball. After a loss, there would be much second-guessing about the instantaneous decisions made on the sidelines by the coaching staff. These meetings reminded me of Grand Rounds at the hospital... but with beer.

The football was exciting, the people were energetic and the beer was good. Attending Cudahy Booster Club meetings provided business and professional contacts and helped grow my medical practice. My Cudahy office patients were good working-class people. Ladish Company, Bucyrus Erie or the Patrick Cudahy meat packing plant employed most of my patients. They were the type of hard working folks I had known well during my childhood and school days. Most of us had had similar aspirations and dreams. We believed if we worked hard or studied hard (or both), there would be a pay-off in the form of economic rewards and lifetime satisfaction. For most of us, this worked out.

Some of my patients were tradesmen with exceptional non-academic skills. These were people who could take a drawing made on a bar napkin and build something that worked. Some of my patients had achieved some higher education and became business or professional people. All my patients had come from the middle and lower economic classes and any success they experienced in their lives had been the result of their own hard work. I understood them and they understood me. Times were good.

The Comfort of Probabilistic Thinking:
Three Terminal Patients and One Lucky Kid

One of the members of the Cudahy Football Booster Club was a forty-something bartender who wanted to own his own place. He had saved his money and rented a space several blocks from my office. His dream was to turn the old corner bar into a neighborhood tavern and sandwich shop. He had been working at his day job and then long hours into the evening to live his dream.

When I saw him in the fall of 1973, he was complaining of fatigue. This could have been easily dismissed as the result of long hours and "getting a little older," but his physical exam revealed he had some unusual bruising that did not seem to be the result of all the manual labor. A blood test in my office showed anemia and a large number of unusual white cells. Dr. Rocco Latorroca, the pathologist at Trinity Hospital, was an excellent physician and a good friend. I asked him to review the hematology slides. The pattern I had observed and diagnosis suspected was confirmed when "probable leukemia" was reported.

Rocco preformed a bone marrow biopsy to confirm the diagnosis. The cell type was not one that responded to chemotherapy. At the time, there was essentially nothing that could be done. Given the stage of the disease at discovery, Rocco believed the man had about six months to live. Like many of my patients, this man was a stoic and had suspected that something serious was wrong for some time. I referred him to a hematologist at the medical school, so he could review his options, but we both knew what the outcome would be. At least he had time to get his affairs in order. As Rocco had predicted, this patient died six months later.

Two other patients also stand out among the many I encountered at that time. A year after this incident, I met a patient who had already run out of time. She was an eighteen-year-old woman who had left home a year before after many years of battling with her father. She was seen on a Monday with a complaint of nosebleeds and unusual bruising. An office exam revealed multiple hematomas that were obviously not the result of trauma. The office blood work showed a severe anemia with very many bizarre white blood cells. She was admitted to Trinity Hospital for evaluation and a transfusion. If there is time, the diagnosis must be established before transfusions are started, but in her case, there was no time. Dr. Latorroca preformed a bone marrow biopsy, and she received several units of packed red blood cells.

By Tuesday afternoon, Rocco had established the diagnosis of an acute form of a rapidly terminal leukemia. When I asked him how long she had, he responded, "She has about a week. She will die shortly of a cerebral hemorrhage and there will be nothing we can do about it." Although she had fallen away from her church, I asked the hospital chaplain and her local parish priest to talk to her and offer any comfort they could.

It took me two days to get her to agree to see her father. This had been a very dysfunctional family, and I felt that if she died before some resolution or we could facilitate at least some degree of closure, the dysfunction for her remaining family members after her passing would get much worse. The father and the rest of her family spent Thursday evening talking together in her hospital room, seemingly reaching some peace. Friday afternoon she suffered a massive cerebral hemorrhage and died.

Shortly after the death of this teenager, a mother brought her two-and-a-half year old daughter to my office for an evaluation. I had been providing check-ups for the child, who had been growing and developing normally. She had learned to walk over a year before the problem developed. After her second birthday, she began to fall to her left while walking. I entered the far end of the hall when the mother and child entered the other end.

The child was walking but falling to her left and bouncing along the corridor wall. As she walked, her left leg appeared weak and lacked coordination. I knew instantly that the child had a tumor on the right side of her brain. Given the child's age, the tumor was probably a highly malignant *astrocytoma*. All I could do was pick up the child and give the mother a hug. I called Children's Hospital and arranged for a neurosurgeon to see the child that day. Even with the best care available at the time, the child died within a year.

These three cases illustrate the deceiving comfort that probabilistic thinking and memory-based decision-making afford the physician. These individuals had very significant terminal conditions that developed rapidly and presented near the end of the course of the disease. Treatment plans for these conditions were well known and not effective. Other medical conditions the patients might have had were insignificant by comparison, and would not necessarily have been evaluated.

In these cases, the probability and the reality matched. Probabilistic thinking and memory-based decision-making worked. Memory-based, global, subjective judgment (i.e., intuition coupled with enough knowledge to be dangerous) works virtually every time for second step or tertiary care from super specialists working in large trauma or specialized medical care centers. Patients come to them with established diagnoses. It is obvious why these physicians have no comprehension regarding the severity of our health care crisis. They only see people who require immediate medically necessary care. They just do not get it. They do not understand the basic needs of the patients on the forefront of medical care who present themselves without a diagnosis.

These super specialists (or "tertiary care" providers) are well trained and experienced in performing the "thing right." As I learned early in my medical career, too frequently doing the "thing right" is trumped by not doing the "right thing." For example, is it the *right thing* to transplant a heart into a known drug addict who has not been rehabilitated and has no social support mechanism? Is it ethical for the surgical transplant team to proceed, knowing the psychiatric and social service consults have determined the patient is not a candidate to receive this limited resource when there are numerous other much more appropriate transplant candidates in dire need? These are not hypothetical questions. This scenario is real and current.

For the docs in the trenches practicing day-to-day medical care, the memory-based probability matches reality most of the time. This is why physicians are able to provide appropriate, medically necessary health care about fifty percent of the time, using the flawed, global, subjective, memory-based decision-making process (also called "intuition"). Our present care delivery system offers little, if any, feedback regarding the quality and appropriateness of all the decisions being made. As a result, it is very difficult to know when unnecessary, ineffective, wasteful care is delivered.

The vast majority of inappropriate and unnecessary care delivered does not usually result in any permanent injury to or death of the patient. The patient may experience discomfort, inconvenience and unnecessary expense, but usually survives the encounter. The human body is so resilient that even when a physician provides inappropriate care, the body will usually heal itself. Such care simply doubles the cost of delivering medical care.

Some of the time doing the *right thing* is just a matter of intuitive dumb luck. For example, a child a little over one year old was brought to my office because of irritability, a runny nose and a slight fever. He was a child I had delivered. Young children pose an especially difficult diagnostic challenge because they are not able to communicate verbally. The physician must be acutely aware of very subtle signs exhibited by the infant or toddler. Behaviors such as pulling or swatting at an ear, what body part moves and what does not, and even the body position held by the child can be very important.

Examination of this child revealed nothing too remarkable aside from some redness in his throat and eardrums. It would have been very easy to diagnose the child as a kid with a cold and send him home with Tylenol samples. Overwhelming probability would drive this diagnosis and plan of treatment. However, something was not right. I do not know if it was the way the child laid on the exam table, or a slight reflex tug I felt in his neck when I picked him up, but I knew this could be more than just a cold.

I called Milwaukee Children's Hospital and arranged for one of the clinic residents to examine the child and have a spinal tap tray ready. An hour later, the child had a stiff neck and white cells in his cerebral spinal fluid. He was immediately admitted and started on intravenous antibiotics. He suffered no complications and recovered completely. Had I sent him home with a fever instruction sheet, he could have easily died of meningitis, or worse, survived with severe brain damage.

Medicine is a Business—Business Decisions Must Be Made

Several years into my solo medical practice, Medicaid instituted a reduced fee schedule for office visits. Medicaid is a state welfare program that funds health care services for those with incomes below a certain level. At various times tax revenues ebb and flow depending on the state of the economy. During tough times, budget cuts are made, usually in health, education and welfare benefits. I do not know if the fee schedule mandated by Medicaid in Wisconsin had anything to do with the establishment of the Federal Health Care Financing Administration (HCFA), but the Medicaid fee schedule had a profound effect on my practice.

The fee for service (FFS) Medicaid rate for a routine office visit (OV) was $6.00 and restrictions were placed on the point of service (POS) for laboratory and X-ray studies. Large clinics with Medicare certified lab, X-ray and day surgery facilities could generate enough FFS reimbursement from these additional services to justify continuing to care for these folks.

At the time, office hourly billing had to generate $70 just to cover business expenses. Without additional cash flow from laboratory tests or X-rays, I would have to see twelve Medicaid enrollees per hour just to generate $72. Such a schedule does not provide enough time for the delivery of quality medical care (one patient every five minutes) and my family could not live on $2.00 per hour.

It was no longer economically feasible to continue serving a significant number of these patients. I stopped billing Medicaid. This is similar to what is happening today with some state and federally funded health care programs.

I had determined I could see one or two patients per hour *pro bono* but more would be too great an economic burden. As Medicare patients were seen, I had to make a determination to officially terminate our professional relationship or select them for ongoing *pro bono* care. I decided that for patients seen for any routine visit, the termination notice could be given at the time of the visit. For patients with ongoing care, *pro bono* services would be continued until the ongoing episode of care ended. I continued providing *pro bono* care to more patients than I could justify from a business standpoint for many years.

I remember one Medicaid enrollee I terminated during a routine visit. She was a healthy 30-something with no apparent family obligations other than caring for herself. She was seen for renewal of her birth control pills but had no other medical problems. She had completed some medical technology training and understood my issue with Medicare.

Talking with me after the office visit, she pointed out the window toward the year-old red Oldsmobile convertible she was driving. I do not know the Medicaid criteria that qualified her for the medical benefit allowing her to see me on the Medicaid plan, and do not want to second guess or criticize overworked public servants, but it seemed to me, she did not need my *pro bono* services. At the time, this "government-run medical care program" seemed well intended. However, somewhere between good intentions and the real world of payment for care, unintended consequences happened.

To supplement my income, I often served as the first assistant for any surgeries on my patients referred to Dr. Sean Keane, one of my favorite orthopedic surgeons. Sean was from Ireland and had immigrated to America. I would perform a pre-op consultation and provide medical clearance for surgery. Sean frequently asked me to do a medical clearance consult prior to surgery on patients admitted through the emergency room.

His technique for assuring the operation would be on the correct knee was to label the patient with permanent marker. He wrote, in three-inch letters, "YES" on the operative site and "NO" on the other knee. He referred a significant number of his post-op patients to a rehabilitation center located several miles north of St. Luke's Hospital. I became associated with this organization and regularly saw patients at the facility.

These patients were generally younger and healthier than the nursing home residents at Willowcrest Care Center, where I served as medical director. Rehabilitation patients were expected to have short stays of intensive physical therapy. Ongoing outpatient therapy was followed by self-care. Sports Medicine was becoming an informal specialty for me. Other physicians were discovering Sports Medicine is a great racket. What could be better than treating young, otherwise healthy people with sprains, strains and minor fractures? Virtually all patients young, well nourished, otherwise healthy patient heal rapidly and are highly motivated to follow physical therapy recommendations. In addition, they are generally willing to pay out-of-pocket for care in excess of their standard indemnity coverage.

I observed that a patient's recovery of normal functioning depended more on the injured patient's psychosocial situation than on the surgeon's skill or the ability and motivational intensity of the best therapists. Patients who were addicted to narcotics, or who had special needs for attention (secondary gain), or those seeking disability status from Worker's Compensation might never improve.

Board Certification Becomes a Necessity, Prescription Drugs a Pitfall

About this time, I became more aware of the political aspects of the business of medicine. I had received my license to practice medicine after passing Part Three of the National Boards in 1969. This was the same year Dr. Pisacano founded the American Board of Family Practice (ABFP). The organization was formed in response to a perceived need for more general practitioners. To achieve this goal, general practice had to be made more attractive to medical school graduates.

When I discovered that a career in radiology was not a good fit, I entered general practice, a medical career that requires no board certification. The ABFP allowed practicing physicians to achieve certification without residency training, if specified continuing medical education (CME) courses were completed and the applicant passed the board certification exam. This process for "grandfathering in" to board certification had a cutoff date during the late 1970s. If I were to become board certified without having to meet the three-year residency requirement, I had to act quickly.

It became obvious that my long-term success as a general practitioner depended on American Board of Family Practice certification. Certification would become a requirement to qualify for hospital staff privileges. As I learned later, Managed Care Organizations (MCOs) required board certification as a key part of the contracting/credentialing process.

Meeting the continuing medical education requirements involved travel, significant expense and time away from the office. Cost was a double-headed dragon. Not only were the CME courses and travel involved expensive, but also time was taken away from the practice and the cash flow it generated. I estimated that the initial American Board of Family Practice certification I achieved in 1977 cost over $30,000.

Certifications had to be renewed through CME attendance and recertification examinations every seven years. I had an impressive certification to hang on my office wall, but I was never able to establish that the educational process and certification ever made any difference in the quality of care delivered. Getting my ticket punched did qualify me to obtain staff privileges with ease and, eventually, to secure my first administrative medical director position. In addition, board certification in a medical specialty was a requirement for board certification in Managed Care.

I should have been more aware of the professional problems that could arise when caring for addicts. I was trained at a time when great advances were being made in medical science, including pharmacology. The DNA double helix structure had been discovered and its description published in 1968. New drugs were put on the market and promoted to physicians at an astounding rate. DuPont's advertising slogan was, "Better things for better living through chemistry."

Many in our military had come home from the Viet Nam War addicted to drugs; some were legal, others were not. It was generally easy to recognize drug-seeking activity when it involved narcotics, but other classes of medications could be addictive without being illegal. Our veterans' problems directly influenced the rules and regulations of state and federal agencies concerning prescriptions written for controlled substances.

During the 1970s and 1980s, prescriptions for appetite suppressants were frequently written for obese patients. Amphetamines and their derivatives were very commonly prescribed. Some of these patients (and the military) used this drug for off-label side effects, principally to increase alertness. Only a small portion of my practice was concerned with monitoring the health status of patients attempting weight loss programs. Any patient I placed on an amphetamine derivative was monitored closely, especially for adverse side effects such as hypertension.

Unfortunately, I *missed the memo* regarding the requirement for psychiatric referral for those patients prescribed these drugs for a specified length of time. One day, I received notification from the state licensing board that they did not approve of my care for a particular patient. They provided me with the regulations involved and a request for medical records. By the time the case was resolved, several years had passed. Alerted now to the issues at hand, I had attended the Continuing Medical Education (CME) course that covered the use of these regulated classes of medications and how to "protect" medical licensure.

With the resolution of the case, the board had issued a sanction requiring me to attend a continuing medical education course and noting I had done so prior to publication of the notice. No suspension or restriction of my medical license was ordered, but I had become older, a little wiser and more humble because of the experience. From that time on, I was exquisitely aware of state and federal regulations and compliance issues. This experience would serve me well in my future adventures.

I voted for Gerald Ford in the1976 Presidential election. The Saturday Night Live parodies of President Ford by Chevy Chase, although extremely funny, did not have a significant influence on the 1976 election. After the fall of Richard Nixon and the country's rejection of the Vietnam War, most people were ready for a change in 1976. Gerald Ford had been a good president, with a few minor foibles. Jimmy Carter seemed to be a good man, but I was very concerned about the election of a "Born Again" Christian to the Presidency.

Our forefathers, being much closer to the religion-based wars that ravaged Europe for centuries, had the good sense to mandate the "Separation of Church and State." I believe Americans concerned about their constitutional freedoms have much more to fear from an American Christian extremist in the White House or on the Supreme Court than any Muslim head of state half way around the world. At least President Carter, like President John F. Kennedy before him, and Teddy Kennedy since, seemed to be able to separate personal religious choices from politics. Jimmy Carter won the election and, during his term, won my respect. He was a good man and a good President.

In 1977, the Health Care Financing Administration (HCFA) was established under the Department of Health Education and Welfare (HEW). This reorganization facilitated HMO financing and development, resulting in a more direct impact on medical practice. In 1980, under President Carter, HEW was split into the Department of Education and the Department of Health and Human Services (HHS). The Health Care Financing Administration (HCFA) has reported to HHS since 2001. Under George W. Bush, Tommy Thompson changed HCFA's name to the Centers for Medicare & Medicaid Services (CMS). "Services" is a much more palatable term than "Financing Agency," don't you think?

CHAPTER 4:
The Managed Care Awakening

In 1978, several years into what had become a very successful medical practice, I was presented with an offer I could not refuse. A general practitioner I had known during my residency at St. Luke's Hospital was leaving practice to retire in Arizona. He was one of the good guys. Dr. King was a no-nonsense GP who practiced quality medicine on the south side of Milwaukee. He owned a one-floor, special purpose medical office building on Oklahoma Avenue near St. Francis Hospital. He had been in practice many years and had a substantial patient following.

Dr. King was retiring to Arizona and motivated to sell his practice. The location, building, office furniture and medical supplies had tangible value. We both realized that patient "good will" and 25¢ would buy anyone a cup of coffee. In fact, if patients stayed with the practice, their paper records would be valuable for their care, but if they left, the costs of copying and mailing records to another physician and their required storage would be a liability. We agreed on a fair price for the building, and I got ready to open in July 1978.

I knew that Dr. King and I would have been compatible as practice partners since we had similar personalities and styles of practice so the transition would not be difficult. However, patients had free choice of physicians, and I would have to earn their respect and loyalty to maintain them. In reality, the office administrative staff and medical personnel, who planned to stay, were the most important assets. His office staff would be staying with the building and the practice. Not only were they extremely competent professionals, they were also very friendly people who knew the patients by name. I am sure many patients stayed with the practice and location because of their relationship with the administrative and medical staff.

When we purchased the office, I applied for staff admitting privileges at St. Francis (now Wheaton Franciscan Health Care) and St. Luke's (now Aurora Health Care). Dr. King had sponsored my application for staff admitting privileges, facilitating the credentialing process by the hospital physician committees.

A year or so after acquiring this second office, I realized working long hours was taking its toll. Admitting patients to three hospitals while attempting to do prenatal care, deliver infants and perform minor surgery made time management difficult. One or two patients admitted to a third hospital can easily add an hour to morning and evening rounds. The economic stress of staffing two offices was hard to carry and became increasingly difficult as malpractice premiums began to rise in the 1970s.

I had arranged some coverage for the Cudahy office when I was not there, but I needed to simplify my life. At this point (in the early 1980s), I gave up deliveries and minor surgery. I stopped admitting patients to St. Luke's Hospital and, after the last patients admitted there had finished their episodes of care, resigned from the staff. My malpractice premiums dropped and my professional life became much more manageable.

The CAT Scanner

Toward the end of the 1970s, I managed a large practice and referred those patients needing specialty care to a group of physicians I felt were the best in the area. My neurology referrals were to a team of two neurologists who were originally from Canada. I am sure their referral pattern analysis showed that I was one of their primary sources. They approached me regarding a partnership in a special purpose CAT scanner (new technology for the time) to be located on the south side of Milwaukee. The business partnership was formed, and the machine was ordered.

This business opportunity had to be seized immediately. In an attempt to control costs, the State of Wisconsin was moving to limit the number of large, expensive machines like scanners by requiring a Certificate of Need (CON). I believe that today we would recognize Wisconsin's attempt to control access as the Canadian method for "rationing." In any event, we could obtain office space and get the machine from General Electric up and running prior to the deadline. My experience with completely remodeling my first office in three weeks paid off.

A small staff and the two neurologists, who read the imaging and produced the reports, managed the facility. Because the technology was new, the absolute value of the test and the clinical indications justifying the procedure were not yet established. I want to believe the referrals I made to my facility were reasonably appropriate. But how could I be sure? There were no universally accepted standards or criteria establishing the medical necessity of the CAT scan. The US Public Task Force on Preventive Health Services had not yet published its report on the effectiveness of screening tests. In fact, to this day CAT scans have never become a justifiable screening test for any medical condition.

The CAT scanner generated enough technical component revenue to produce a small profit. After several years, the technology had advanced and larger, more powerful machines had been installed in the hospitals. Three years later, our facility was sold to one of the hospitals where the neurologists practiced. The partnership was dissolved. The location was used as an outpatient satellite office, managed by the hospital, for a number of years. It was finally closed after a technology upgrade to the hospital based systems.

The outcomes of this project taught me two important lessons. First, it is impossible to control costs through restricting the latest medical technology from an administrative level. The State of Wisconsin's attempt at rationing health care through the Certificate of Need restriction was not effective. The regulators were no match for well-organized hospital systems and their thousands of supportive patients. The wants and desires of the medical staff and their patients are impossible for hospital administrators or state regulators to block. As long as the administrators and their accountants determined that a new technology can generate profit, high-tech, expensive medical machinery will be installed.

Second, it is easy for medical practitioners to succumb to costly and unnecessary testing when the machinery has a lot of bells and whistles and maps out data in full color images. Standards of practice and rigorous criteria must be implemented for physicians to work towards controlling costs. It wasn't until the 1990s that the utilization review departments of HMOs would effectively implement the criteria and standards that were ultimately developed. It wasn't until that same decade that HMOs enrolled enough patients and increased their market share such that they could actually impact utilization and slow the increasing cost of care resulting from the delivery of unnecessary services. The cost of our medical-industrial complex outpaced inflation as high tech medical care expanded. Despite the full color images of our diseases, quality of care failed to improve.

Lament for my Uncle Allan

One summer during the late 1970s, Aunt Elaine and her husband Allan returned to Milwaukee for a family visit. I invited them to a social event held on the grounds of South Shore Yacht Club in early June. I remember the conversation with Uncle Allan as if it happened yesterday. The sky was deep blue and a cool southeast breeze moderated the effects of the warm afternoon sun as we sat around a picnic bench near the front dock. He told me he had been diagnosed with coronary artery disease and would be going back to Detroit to have revascularization surgery in early July. His surgery would be done at the university hospital.

There have been a few times over the years when I have seen a skull and crossbones as I've looked into a person's eyes (metaphorically, of course, since I am not subject to hallucinations). With Uncle Allan, a sense of apprehension and foreboding come over me. I understood the bad things that can happen to patients in a university hospital in July, just after the residents rotate—I had experienced rotations during my residency when things did not run smoothly with brand new and unpracticed medical teams that did not yet work together well. I also knew that complication rates varied wildly between institutions, and that cardiac surgery at a large private institution with a mature, well-trained team of physicians, nurses, anesthesiologists and other professionals usually produced better outcomes than county or university settings.

Because I had been a resident at St. Luke's Hospital in Milwaukee, I had the opportunity to observe the cardiac surgery teams in action from an insider's perspective. I wanted to tell my Uncle to come to Milwaukee and St. Luke's Hospital for his surgery, but I held my tongue, smiled and wished him good luck with his care in Detroit. I think of myself as very objective, and there are good reasons why physicians should not treat or advise family members—for example, judgment may become clouded when emotion is a factor. After all, the probability of a bad outcome at the university hospital was only a small percent. I believed St. Luke's Hospital could provide better care and a better chance at a good outcome, but there are no guarantees where high tech medical care is concerned. I did not push for the change of venue to St. Luke's Hospital. It may not have mattered anyway.

Uncle Allan returned to Detroit and had surgery early that July. The operation was a success, but he developed an infection several days later. He never made it out of the hospital alive. He suffered a painful, protracted, progressive infection in his chest wall, rib cage and heart for six weeks. He died in August. The cause of death was septicemia, commonly known as "blood poisoning," from a nosocomial (hospital-based) infection.

I never reviewed his medical records, so I did not know if the surgery was medically necessary or if heart medication would have been equally effective. I do not know if the hospital ever evaluated my Uncle's death to determine if the surgical procedure was appropriately done (doing the "thing right") or if the surgery was necessary (doing the "right thing"). I did not know the postoperative infection rate of the hospital or of the surgical team doing cardiac revascularization, although I do know that post-op infections are usually caused by poor sterile technique. Had a report card system been in place at that time, I believe I could have discussed his choices with him objectively. This might have led to a very different ending to the story.

Cost, Quality and Competition

Some politicians and economists believe the pressures of our capitalist marketplace, if allowed to function with minimal regulatory interference, will drive cost down and improve quality. This approach to our health care crisis might actually work if health care followed the principle of supply and demand. If health care functioned like a commodity market, competition might drive down cost while improving quality, but health care is not a commodity... yet. The American patient's demand for health related services is insatiable. In Metropolitan Statistical Areas (MSAs) with an excess supply of physicians, cost and the frequency of unnecessary care are higher. Excessive demand drives costs up and an excess supply of providers makes things worse.

America's health care costs began skyrocketing during the 1970s, as health care organizations converted to for-profit status. For-profit corporations now dominate our medical-industrial complex. In my opinion, competition in our present health care delivery system is between a few large for-profit corporations—smaller providers (like my solo practice) can no longer compete against them. These gigantic organizations are in the business of making money, not providing health care. For Americans with relatively large amounts of disposable income (compared to many other nations), public records, financial reports and stockbrokers provide reliable information facilitating the selection of the best health care corporation for your health care investment dollars. The winners in this game are those who create the greatest profit for their shareholders and largest bonuses for their executives. The quality of care delivered to patients is never measured and not a concern. I do not point this out to make a moral judgment or define our for-profit health care delivery system as good or bad. Our medical-industrial complex is a product of the American capitalist economic system. It is what it is and will not change significantly while profit rules and health care is considered a privilege.

The *Dartmouth Atlas* (www.dartmouthatlas.org) is an excellent source for academicians researching where dollars are spent in the medical-industrial complex. It also provides insight regarding the disparity in health care between geographic locations. The Dartmouth Atlas is a scoreboard of sorts and implies that the quality of care is variable. It does not offer provider-specific information about the quality of care any single institution or physician delivers.

For competition to improve the quality of health care services while reducing costs, the parameters of the competition must be well defined. Basic microeconomics explain that for supply and demand to function properly, consumers must have all information available to them to make rational, intelligent decisions. In the real world, consumers are not provided the key data required to make competition in the marketplace reflect real demand. American consumers need specific information about each physician and institution to make more intelligent decisions. This data is available, although not publicly, and has been for forty years. Advances in information technology made cost and quality data available in the claims systems of insurance companies. Reports could have been published to show specific hospital and physician complication rates. The cost of care by hospital and physician for key high dollar diseases could have been made public. It was not done when it was first possible, and it is not being done now.

The good, the bad and the ugly *must* be made public. For competition to drive cost and quality, physician and hospital cost, outcome, complication and error rates must be published. A consumer driven health care system will not work until consumers know the quality of the care they are buying. Competition over which for-profit insurance company saves the consumer a dollar here and there is meaningless.

The Dawn of the Managed Care Age in Milwaukee

At the end of the 1970s, Managed Care Organizations (MCOs) and Health Maintenance Organizations (HMOs) finally started to have an impact in Milwaukee. Although the effect on my practice was minimal, I could see the future. As a solo practitioner, I was not a member of any managed care panel and therefore had no contact with any insurance utilization review department. I was not required to call any review organization to obtain authorization for any care I ordered or referral I made.

A small trickle of patients with new HMO insurance policies requested transfer of their records to large clinics. I discussed this with many patients, who said that they were satisfied with my staff and my care; however, their employers had offered options for their health insurance—the available HMO plan cost less and included better benefits than their standard indemnity coverage.

I was to learn much later that the price on a doctor's head was $25. In other words, if the worker could save $25 per month, the patient would leave their family physician in exchange for a different primary care provider listed on the new health care plan's network. To save network development costs, Managed Care Organizations (MCOs) only establish contracts with larger clinics, not solo practitioners. This was nothing personal—it was smart business. In addition, large clinics could offer a package deal of primary care physicians alongside many specialists with one stroke of the pen. Clinic administration could facilitate communication with and education of clinic physicians regarding specific contract requirements and general managed care principles.

Many hospital administrations built large office complexes on or near the grounds and offered physician office space at lower rental rates than those prevailing in the area. They understood that their future success depended on the success of their staff physicians. The physicians renting these spaces were independent of the hospital across the street, but the relationship was tight. This owner/renter contract functioned like a very loosely managed group practice medical clinic.

Hospital administrators knew Managed Care Organizations meant trouble for their business operations and bottom line. I have to believe that most Milwaukee hospital administrators were studying the laws and federal regulations enhancing the development of managed care. They understood that their future success depended on the success of their staff physicians. The development of Physician-Hospital Organizations (PHOs) could provide administrators some control of the market. However, the financial success of hospitals and their administrators depend on keeping their staff physicians happy. At the time, practicing physicians were fearful about the managed care menace. The development of PHOs would take several years.

The administrators soon learned that low office rental rates and convenience would not necessarily be enough to ensure loyalty or compliance. A PHO would be an ideal relationship to develop only if the physicians were able to conceptualize the business side of medicine. However, organizing a large group of very independent minded, anti-HMO physicians was a formidable task. The problems of influencing the direction and decisions of the tenant independent practitioners are similar to the problems of cat herders. Herding cats may be easier. The hospital administrators, as property owners, have much less influence than the administrators of large clinics (e.g., Milwaukee, Mayo Brothers, Cleveland, Dartmouth-Hitchcock, etc.) where the physicians function as employees.

As a solo practitioner at this time, I was still relatively unaffected by these machinations. Solo and small partnership practices would have to wait for the MCOs, HMOs and insurance companies to develop the infrastructure to contract and service these practices in widespread locations. I understood the delay but did not like waiting until the future happened to me. However, I was very busy practicing medicine so my time was limited, and I really did not know what I could do about this looming challenge.

The Awakening: 1979

At a St. Francis Hospital staff meeting in 1979, a physician from Intergroup in Chicago delivered a presentation explaining the contractual relationship his organization had with CNA Insurance and their HMO product. Prior to this presentation, I had no firsthand knowledge and no understanding of managed care or Health Maintenance Organizations. I also did not really understand standard indemnity health insurance even though I was purchasing it for my family and my employees.

National insurance companies such as CNA, Metropolitan, Prudential and others have their home offices in a central location nationally, but each state regulates insurance products marketed within its borders making state offices extremely important. Intergroup was an association of a large number of independent Chicago physician practices that formed a loose association for contracting with CNA Insurance Company of Illinois to offer managed care plans to large employers. A group of medical professionals made up of solo practitioners, partnerships and clinics is called an "Independent Practice Association" or IPA. The contractual relationship between the two entities formed "CNA-Intergroup," a federally qualified HMO.

Federal law mandated that any business that employed over twenty-five workers had to offer a "dual option" including an HMO if one were available. CNA-Intergroup had been formed to take advantage of this mandate in the Chicago area. This company allowed physicians in solo practices or small partnerships to compete with the large clinic HMOs.

The presenter delivered a very clear, concise explanation of the essential differences between indemnity insurance companies and Health Maintenance Organizations (HMOs). Insurance companies primarily focus on managing financial risk. Because they manage financial risk for medical care, they are called "indemnity" companies. Indemnity insurance companies are known as "payers," because they pay health care claims. The financial risk for the cost of covered benefits is spread across all employees of the employer and transferred to the insurance company through premium payments. Health care cost risk management is the business focus of indemnity insurance.

The patients covered by the indemnity insurance company are known as the "insureds." The employers of these insureds purchase health care on behalf of their employees. Because of this financial reality, employers are sometimes called "purchasers." In reality, the employers are really the intermediaries that establish the contractual relationship between the insured worker and their indemnity insurance company. The presenter pointed out there is no contractual relationship between the indemnity insurance company and the medical community.

The presenter contrasted the financial risk management model of indemnity insurance with the preventive care and health improvement model of managed care. There is a contractual relationship between the health care plan and the physicians. The primary focus of the Managed Care Organization (MCO) is on managing appropriate, effective efficient health care. The contract they enter establishes some shared financial risk management between the MCO and the primary care physicians. This transfer of financial risk for patient care is limited and well defined. This means the doctors have some skin in the game. They are no longer only spending other people's money (OPM).

The employer purchases health care coverage on behalf of the employee, as in the indemnity insurance model. The health care financing model is referred to as a Health Care Plan rather than a Health Insurance Policy. The covered employee is a *member* of a plan rather than an *insured* of an insurance company. Medical caregivers in the health care plan are called service *providers*. The essential difference is the presence of a contractual relationship between the member, provider and health care plan.

The HMO developed a "gatekeeper" model in order to provide the most effective care using resources most efficiently. Patients first see the general practitioner—the gatekeeper—who can take care of most basic needs and recognize the need for any particular specialist. The gatekeeper or Primary Care Provider (PCP) now includes family practice, pediatrics, OB/Gyn and some internists. It makes great logical sense to take care of ourselves this way. The Primary Care Provider (PCP) has a broad, general knowledge of disease states and anatomical systems, and can refer any conditions requiring more detailed examination and more complex treatment to the most appropriate specialist. Doctor-to-doctor patient referrals are generally expedited saving time for the patient. In addition, most tertiary care specialists will not accept patients without screening/evaluation and referral by a primary care physician. Patients frequently do not benefit by seeking specialty care directly because "to a guy with a hammer, everything looks like a nail." In other words, a heart specialist may not be looking at the endocrine system for the root of the problem or for the solution. In addition, the specialist will be more costly and will not always produce an effective outcome.

The HMO gatekeeper model was additionally designed to give the physicians an investment in keeping their assigned population of patients healthy and provide the tools to do so. The plan members have benefits that exceed those of standard indemnity insurance policies, including preventive care, wellness and education. These incentives drive the provision of cost-effective, quality health care to best manage patient problems. This model not only places control of primary care services with the PCP, it also requires the PCP to authorize referrals to specialists. Prior evaluation of a patient's problem by the primary care doctor would assure the most efficient triage to the most appropriate specialist.

With shared risk comes shared reward. If unnecessary medical care were avoided, the primary care provider shared in the savings. The HMO concept of giving the primary care physician the financial resources, limited financial risk and potential financial reward for delivering quality care to a population of patients made perfect sense to me.

The presenter also brought a business perspective to the economics of health care financing. Worker's wages, worker compensation, health insurance, disability insurance and unemployment coverage are all direct costs of labor to the employer. Health care coverage is a large portion of this cost. The reader must understand the cost of health care coverage is a large portion of the cost of labor and therefore comes indirectly out of the employee's pocket. Keep in mind, the employee is ultimately the purchaser of health care coverage.

I saw the light. I was one of the few physicians at the meeting who got the message and understood the cost containment and quality improvement implications of the gatekeeper model. I was ready to organize a community of like-minded medical care providers. If our local physicians formed such an IPA, we could contract with any insurance company (claims payer) that wanted to offer federally qualified managed care plans. This would give the primary care solo and small partnership physicians on the south side of Milwaukee the vehicle to compete with the large HMOs.

The local provider relations representative, Michael M., accompanied the physician presenter. I asked Michael for additional information; he and CNA Insurance provided a complete package for the practitioner who wished to establish an IPA. It was a cookbook for the development of an Independent Practice Association.

South Shore IPA: 1980

In 1980, under President Jimmy Carter, the Health Care Financing Administration (HCFA) was placed under the newly created Department of Health and Human Services. Most physicians viewed additional oversight by government bureaucrats as more interference with the practice of medicine and a greater administrative burden. I did not know if this federal administrative reorganization was a good or bad thing for medicine. I did understand that the American health care system required some degree of oversight, and physicians needed to be leading the parade, not digging in our heels while being dragged to a future beyond our control.

I filed "South Shore IPA Inc." with the State of Wisconsin. The generic CNA physician provider contracts were modified so that South Shore IPA held the physician contracts. The contract between CNA and South Shore IPA was modified, eliminating the exclusive CNA clause. This would allow the IPA to negotiate and contract with payers other than CNA.

I began recruiting physicians for South Shore IPA from the Trinity and St. Francis hospitals and setting up credentialing and quality improvement committees. I recruited 130 doctors, a sufficient number of primary care and specialty physicians over a broad enough geographical area to meet the requirements of federal qualification. CNA held a license to sell health insurance products in Wisconsin. With our IPA network contracted, they became a federally qualified HMO poised to market their health care plan.

Organized medicine had been on the wrong side of every progressive social issue in the twentieth century and needed to be taking the lead on health care reform. I believed a private solution to rising medical costs, facilitated by appropriate legislation, was achievable through the development of Managed Care Organizations (MCOs) and Health Maintenance Organizations (HMOs).

Prior to marketing their HMO product in Milwaukee, CNA sold their HMO products and license to Maxicare, a California HMO. Insiders affectionately knew this organization as the "Pam and Fred show." I would learn later that it is more profitable to build and sell a network of physicians than to operate the health care plan (herd the cats) once it is organized.

From 1980 through the summer of 1985, I was the part-time medical director for South Shore IPA and a full-time family medicine practitioner in solo practice. The obligations and pressures of operating a small business and solo practice remained constant as the time I spent on IPA administration grew. As the medical director, I did the physician recruitment and chaired the mandated Credentials, Peer Review and Quality Assurance Committees. The IPA evolved with the pressures of the market place and variable practice patterns of contracted physicians.

Maxicare marketed their federally qualified HMO in the local marketplace and determined the final monthly price for the health care plan. The actuaries at Maxicare, using their crystal balls, allocated the health care plan premium to a primary care fund (about 20 percent), a specialty fund (about 20 percent), a hospitalization fund (about 50 percent) and the administrative fee (about 10 percent). The IPA primary care fund amounted to approximately $21 per enrollee per month.

This fund covered services delivered or ordered by the PCP gatekeeper selected by the member. All outpatient laboratory tests and X-rays ordered by the PCP were paid from the primary care fund, according to the negotiated FFS billing schedule. By contrast, the IPA gatekeeper primary care providers agreed to a floating fee schedule, loosely based on the Medicare relative value scale, for hospital in-patient and office outpatient visits. If there were a shortfall in the money allocated to the primary care fund (if the total PCP charges exceeded the monthly funding), fees for services were reduced, so the IPA would remain solvent. Later, during my corporate life, I would learn a great deal about the dangers of the term "allocation": allocation works much better if the entity doing the allocating also bears the risk.

Specialists listed on the referral panel submitted claims to Maxicare that complied with a standard contractual fee schedule. Specialists were not at risk for any shortfalls, but their fee schedule essentially matched that of Medicare. Fifty percent of any "surplus" in the specialty fund allocation was to be shared with the IPA.

Maxicare provided reinsurance for individual member losses over $100,000 per annum. This is like the umbrella liability policy some people carry on their auto and home insurance. Any IPA specialty fund savings would be used to compensate the PCP doctors based on their individual portion of total IPA submitted claims. Any specialty fund surplus remaining after paying the IPA administrative fees and paying primary care gatekeeper physician fees would apply to PCP bonuses for delivery of quality care.

The physician Quality Assurance Committee would determine the methodology for assessing quality and distribution of quality bonuses. All physicians were prohibited, by contract, from "balance billing" a member/patient for any additional amount above the agreed fee for IPA reimbursement.

I never received a salary or any other form of compensation for my work organizing or managing any aspect of South Shore IPA. The Association did have one employee (Sue Giamo) who processed the claims for the specialty providers. During the five years I managed South Shore IPA, the only expenses were office supplies and Sue's hourly wage. She occupied a desk in my medical office record room. No fees (commonly called "charge back") were ever collected from the IPA for this office space. The IPA administrative expenses were kept extremely low.

The design of the primary care gatekeeper managed health care plan was based on several principles and assumptions. Maxicare set the expense ratios and fund allocations for this gatekeeper model based on actuarial guidelines adjusted for Milwaukee. A central record-keeping site was assumed to result in administrative cost savings. The PCP was assumed to have a reasonable understanding of appropriate medical care. This medical provider was expected to avoid providing or ordering care that was not medically necessary.

In this model, the patient accesses the delivery system through the gatekeeper, who either provides primary care services or coordinates referrals for all other care. With a broad, general knowledge of medicine, the PCP gatekeeper is the most qualified to triage patients efficiently. This knowledge facilitates referral of the patient to the most appropriate setting and specialty physician. Specialists more appropriately manage more complex care delivery. Today, some people refer to this model as "Patient-Centered Medical Home."

The IPA was paid a monthly fee called *capitation* for each assigned member. This global capitated payment for primary care services transferred significant financial risk from Maxicare to the physicians for the services defined in the primary care fund. The term *"capitation"* comes from the Latin word for head. The Roman Army paid their physicians a fee per head to care for their centurions. My year of high school Latin finally paid off.

Capitation and population management may date back to ancient China. Physicians were paid based on the population they served, not the services performed. Of course, when the plague came to the Provence and killed a large percentage of the population, the Emperor had the physicians executed—a very effective incentive for public health officials to do their best to keep the population under their management healthy.

In this gatekeeper model, the PCP was required to authorize member visits to plan specialists. The specialists were paid the negotiated fee for services they provided, and were at no financial risk for the care they delivered. The IPA paid specialist and consultant fees from the Specialty Fund held by Maxicare. The financial success of the South Shore IPA depended on the primary care doctors making sound medical judgments in order to deliver appropriate, effective and efficient care. However, the determination of what care will be delivered is not the sole prerogative of the physician. The patient's medically necessary needs are primary, but their wants and desires virtually always have some influence on medical judgments.

Maxicare's actuaries determined the amount allocated to this fund each month. The amount allocated to the specialty fund per member per month (the monthly capitation) was about twenty dollars. Because the specialists had no risk, they had no reward. In theory, if the gatekeeper PCP's made only medically necessary specialty referrals and resisted at least 20 percent of member requests for unnecessary referrals, the specialty allocation would have excess funds. Because any excess in this allocation would be the result of appropriate cost containment decisions made by the PCPs, a portion would flow back into the primary care allocation to make up for any shortfalls. If additional dollars remained at the end of the year, the IPA committees could consider quality care bonuses.

In the real world, most of the physicians did not attempt to consider medical necessity when making referrals for high-tech, expensive testing or specialty evaluation. Few PCPs resisted any patient's push for irrational or unnecessary medical services. The amount of care delivered continued to exceed the care that was medically necessary and the billed cost of care exceeded the dollars allocated to the funds.

Sue Giamo, the only IPA employee, processed claims for the IPA primary care providers and specialist panel physicians. Maxicare produced complete financial reports on a monthly basis. As medical director, I reviewed these financial statements and presented them to the physicians at the monthly IPA meetings. The physicians began to understand the financial impact of their medical decisions. However, it was obvious to several members of the board and to me that the group continued to think in terms of fee-for-service (FFS) piecework medical care delivery.

Maxicare grew slowly over the next several years, enrolling thousands of members into the plan. The viability of the plan depended on the physician providers' capability to differentiate medically necessary care from unnecessary services. The reimbursements to the various funds set by the corporate actuaries should have been adequate to cover all the medical expenses of the enrollees. If the contracted providers practiced common sense, applied medicine conservatively and eliminated as much unnecessary care as possible, quality bonuses should have become a reality. Common sense and moderation never prevailed.

Most of the IPA physicians continued to spend other people's money like drunken sailors. Although the doctors had some skin in the game through positive and negative incentives for proper risk management, most were never able to rid themselves of their piecework, FFS mindset. Although physician reimbursement was based on fees charged, the budget for the IPA was based on a per-member, per-month capitation. Maxicare determined the allocation of premium dollars in the form of capitation to the various IPA funds.

The IPA was capitated and primary care providers' fees were paid in proportion to dollars in the fund at the end of the month. If the fund had only 90 percent of the dollars needed to pay all the FFS charges submitted by the PCPs, the doctors were paid 90 percent of their billed charges. The physician was not allowed to bill the patient for the balance.

As Maxicare sold HMO coverage to Wisconsin employers, the plan grew to tens of thousands of members. As the plan grew, so did the shortfalls and cuts to physician reimbursement. In response to fee reductions, IPA physicians billed more services to make up for the shortfall. The original agreement between the IPA and Maxicare was not sustainable, and would soon fall apart.

The Gatekeeper HMO Model

Seven hundred members had selected me as their PCP by January 1985. By June 1985, my practice was assigned over 900 Maxicare members. The practice had a statistical cross section of patients. This large number assured that the Maxicare patients were of average health status and carried an average disease load. Some of my assigned folks had serious medical problems but most were of very average health, making the system very workable.

The IPA was funded for all assigned members including those who never got sick and never sought medical care from their primary care provider (PCP). The PCPs saw only the portion of their total assigned membership that accessed care at their offices. The doctors provided services to the patients they treated for the negotiated Maxicare FFS payment schedule. The Maxicare actuaries built the delivery of a modest amount of unnecessary care, but the risk of financial loss through overutilization was no longer solely the payer's problem— the insurance company was not the only money in the game. The risk-sharing model assured that the providers—the doctors—had a great deal of skin in the game as well. Decisions made by the physicians determined whether black or red ink flowed to the bottom line. Funding of quality bonuses should have been possible, but it never happened.

Differentiating "medically necessary" from "not medically necessary" care is not difficult for the extreme ends of the patient complaint or problem spectrum. Making appropriate decisions in the middle ground is much more difficult. Help with these difficult decisions was becoming available. Various professional medical organizations had begun distributing standards of care developed through application of the science of clinical epidemiology. These criteria and standards, including scientifically sound, easy-to-follow checklists, would facilitate making decisions resulting in reducing unnecessary services. Physicians needed to adjust their practice and habits to apply these standards when they treated their patients to assure delivery of quality care and black ink to the bottom line.

Doing the "right thing" for the patient in real time should be the easy part. Nevertheless, the physician decision-making process is only half the equation. Patient expectations and demands also drive the cost of care. Patients frequently have unrealistic expectations about the capability of modern medicine. Few patients understand the scientific basis for determining the difference between necessary and unnecessary care. Patients find reconciling their desires and wants with what they need, or what modern medical care can do for them, very difficult. If patients did understand the difference, they would make fewer demands for unnecessary medical care.

We should not consider patients "wise consumers" of medical care, nor should we expect patients to know the difference between necessary and unnecessary care. They generally know very little about the science of medicine and less about what works and what does not. Most have blind faith in their doctors' decisions or know they can push their physicians to order almost anything they demand. Most physicians will not risk losing the "customer" by refusing to order the requested unnecessary service or unnecessary consultation. Most physicians will not spend the time or effort to educate the patient. There is no fee for this service. Many physicians, in spite of their education, training and experience, practice medicine as if they do not understand medical necessity.

When health care funding is through for-profit indemnity insurance companies using the fee-for-service reimbursement methodology, both the patient and the physician perceive they are spending other people's money. A capitated PCP, managing a population of HMO patients, has some financial risk for the care ordered. The physician has an incentive to educate patients who have unrealistic expectations or make demands for unnecessary services.

During this time, two patient referral requests stand out in my memory. A woman I saw in my office on a first visit complained of psychological stress resulting from a financial situation. She wanted a referral for psychotherapy but needed to see a financial counselor. Clearly, financial counseling was not a covered benefit of her health care plan. Her financial problems were not severe and her stress could have been easily managed in a primary care setting. She was not a danger to herself or others, but her request was very unusual and disturbing.

She demanded an authorization referral to see her out of network "Christian psychologist." The Maxicare provider network listed two psychiatrists. I knew the panel psychiatrists well. They received all my referrals, regardless of the patient's insurance or health care plan. I knew they were both Jewish. I did not know if this patient was simply anti-Semitic or if she believed Christian providers have powers beyond the ordinary. Either way, she was unreceptive to seeking counseling from two very qualified professionals who might have helped her, regardless of their religious background.

There was no point attempting a rational discussion with this patient. I had been there and done that during my internship when I had to watch the young mother of two bleed to death because her religion forbade transfusion.

I told this patient I could approve a referral to a Maxicare panel psychiatrist, but if she wanted to see an out of network provider, she would need to pay for all visits out-of-pocket. These were the days before partial payment for out of network, non-emergent care.

I do not remember if she transferred to another Maxicare PCP or selected another insurance plan, but I never saw her again. This encounter affirmed my belief that the effect of religious institutions must be neutral in the practice of medicine and, by extension, out of government where laws and regulations affecting medical science and the design of health care plans are made. Too many bad decisions are made when religious doctrine is allowed to skew the process. Our Founding Fathers were correct in separating church and state. I can only hope our present elected officials have the wisdom to separate religion and the medical care delivery system.

Learning to Listen: The First Step Towards the Vision

The referral request made by another patient would have a small immediate but very profound long-term effect on me. She and her pre-teen son were seen on an initial visit. Her care would be routine and uncomplicated. She additionally wanted a referral to an endocrinologist for her diabetic son. I cared for many diabetic patients in my practice as outpatients. I had treated patients with a diabetic crisis in the hospital. I felt reasonably knowledgeable regarding diabetes and believed I was competent to treat her son as an outpatient in my office.

When I told her I could treat her son and did not think the referral was necessary, she asked me if I knew the difference between Type I and Type II diabetes. I quickly got over the insult of this mere mortal woman questioning my skill, knowledge and authority as a male physician (and minor deity). I assured her I understood it and returned the question—did *she* know the difference between Type I and Type II Diabetes.

As she talked and I listened, it became clear that she probably knew as much about diabetes as I did. In addition, she had the equivalent of a Ph.D. in the disease specifically as it affected her son and was intimately knowledgeable about the psychosocial impact diabetes had on him and the family over his entire life. She was the expert on the uniqueness of her son. I was just the guy empowered by the state licensing board to diagnose and treat patients.

I understood that Maxicare, through capitation, had given me control of significant funding to manage the care of my population of patients. I could deliver quality care to most of my diabetic patients. If referral to the endocrinologist for this special case resulted in just marginally better control of the disease for this child, he would be healthier.

Longer-term, his total health care costs would be lower. Diabetes is a complicated disease and patients require significant time at every office visit to adequately manage their care. By doing what his mother asked, the quality of his care would improve and the costs for his care would ultimately be lower. This encounter was a turning point in my career, and set me on the path towards what ultimately would become my vision for health care, and the reason I am writing this book. I authorized the referral. I believed the decision was appropriate at the time, and I still do. It would be years before I understood the wisdom of this mother and the profound positive quality impact managing groups of individuals with certain diseases provides. It turned out capitation is an effective financial foundation for both the gatekeeper model and for compensating teams of providers that manage the health care of populations of patients with specific high cost disease processes.

Fee-For-Service Payment—The Enemy of Quality Care

At that time, I felt confident that I understood health maintenance and managing care because of my experience with these patients and my belief in the HMO concept of health care delivery. I continued to learn new things about practicing medicine under the HMO model through patients like those described above. My practice style and my practice patterns fit well into the parameters set by Maxicare. A few of us could offer what I believed to be quality care at a lower cost, although many fellow providers in our group were not able to achieve the goal of cost-effective quality care. The plan-wide projected IPA cost reductions never happened. The structural model was correct, but the human implementation failed.

Most physicians were not able to make the adjustment from the FFS free-for-all spending model to the HMO/MCO model that required the conscious awareness of medical necessity and the cost of care. Individual self-interest, driven by FFS reimbursement, ruled the system. Many IPA physicians continued their habitual excessive referral practice patterns for tests and specialty services. The rate of unnecessary referrals and the amount of unnecessary care overwhelmed the conservative pricing model.

An additional problem with this model: the specialists had no financial risk and were paid based on their contracted FFS schedule. Other than the negotiated fee reductions, they never absorbed additional losses—they had no skin in the game. The primary care fund allocation was never enough to cover 100 percent of the fees submitted by the PCPs.

The IPA struggled financially for several years. Most months, fees had to be cut by several percentage points. Primary care physicians began to drop out of the panel as their reimbursements dropped. The relationship between South Shore IPA and Maxicare required restructuring. At the end, after payment of all laboratory, X-ray and specialty referral costs, the PCPs were paid about twenty-five cents on the dollar for their office visits. As they dropped out, their patients were allowed to select one of the remaining physicians.

The final ten physicians with the majority of the enrollment agreed to go forward with a modified reimbursement methodology. The capitated IPA primary care fund pool was eliminated. Each PCP was allocated an individual practice fund based on a per-member, per-month capitation. All professional services and all outpatient laboratory and X-ray care were paid from this fund. Authorized specialty care, outpatient laboratory and X-rays were paid first. Then the PCP fees were paid. At the end of the contract year, any excess dollars would be split between Maxicare and the PCP managing his individual care fund.

The physicians continuing their relationship with Maxicare and the IPA understood the original system was an intermediate step from fee-for-service (FFS) reimbursement toward capitation. They knew that the success of the original larger group had depended on relying on a majority of providers to practice cost-effective, quality medical care. They also knew that excessive referrals for unnecessary services by some physicians had brought the IPA to its knees.

I had experience with these unfettered costs as medical care was spinning out of control and knew some form of managed care was the answer. I had seen the light and wanted to carry it forward, but my efforts seemed to be like a candle in the wind. I needed to do more.

The 1984 Presidential election was essentially a walk through the park for Ronald Reagan. Walter Mondale seemed to be an honorable man, but not a viable contender. I liked the GOP's program of low taxes and private sector growth. I voted for President Reagan, who won in 49 out of 50 states. It was a landslide. I was not sure "supply side Reaganomics" made sound economic policy for the country but I knew, because of my income bracket, voodoo economics would be good for my family.

Maxicare Version Two and Moving On

December 31, 1984, marked the end of the first generation IPA contract with Maxicare. The new financial arrangement with the remaining "gang of ten" (the second iteration of Maxicare) began January 1, 1985. By the end of 1984, my practice included about 700 Maxicare enrollees. This number would increase to 900 by the end of June 1985. New members were encouraged to visit their chosen PCP's office to get to know their new doctor and have their medical records transferred. The physicians were to assess the patient's medical and psychosocial needs. Medical record transfer requests were executed. Comprehensive care management, rather than incident-based medical practice, would begin.

The gatekeeper PCP owns both the resources and some of the financial risk for managing primary and specialty care for a defined group of patients. Each PCP in our Maxicare "gang of ten" had a significant number of enrollees (the population) and a significant allocation of money (capitation) to provide all necessary and even a little bit of unnecessary care. The relatively large number of members assigned to each practice favored a statistically average risk (or cost per patient) and had the viability of a population management model. My practice illustrates these concepts.

Using round numbers, capitation per member for my Maxicare primary care fund totaled about $21,000 per month or approximately $252,000 per annum. All primary care services, outpatient laboratory and X-ray imaging were paid from this fund. My office had the laboratory, ECG and X-ray facilities to accommodate most medically necessary services defined as primary care. I also performed minor office surgery and some simple suturing. As a result, my referral authorization for care outside my office was minimized. The primary care services provided in my office consumed the entire Maxicare primary care allocation fund. Maxicare allocated an additional $21,000 per month or $252,000 per annum to my specialty capitation fund. For 1985, the primary care fund plus the specialty capitation fund totaled about $504,000 in resources available to manage the health, preventive care, and disease processes for my assigned population. This fund paid for all specialist care, including consultations and surgical procedures, whether inpatient or outpatient. I provided most medical services in my office and authorized referrals to specialists for medically necessary care only. If this strategy were successful, by the end of 1985 my specialty fund should have shown a surplus.

During the first half of the year, by providing most routine and uncomplicated services in my office, I used all the money available in my primary care fund. However, my specialty care fund had a $37,000 reserve. Looking at it another way, within a total budget of $252,000 for six months (half of the primary care fund and half of the specialty care fund for the year) I managed all the medical care required for a population of 900 for a total cost of $210,000. I saved $37,000 or 14.7 percent of the actuarially projected cost of managing this population for six months by practicing common sense medicine.

Putting this number into today's context, if all physicians in America followed conservative, patient-centered, practice patterns our present health care expenditure of $2.5 trillion[4] could be cut by 14.7 percent or $366 billion. That is billion with a "B" and it is a yearly cost reduction.

Keep in mind that I was practicing in a primary care, gatekeeper, capitated, managed care model. The financial incentives were aligned with cost-effective quality care. There was no bureaucratic oversight or review. Nevertheless, the majority of the original South Shore IPA primary care providers could not shift away from FFS piecework reimbursement to payment through capitation for managing a population of patients. It may be extremely difficult for most physicians to transition from an incident-based medical practice style to patient-centered medical management, but changing this paradigm is necessary to control our skyrocketing medical costs.

The contract with Maxicare stated the primary care provider would receive half the dollars remaining in the capitated funds as a bonus for practicing cost-effective medicine. I had saved $37,000 in the first six months and was on track to double that by the end of the year. If I continued to practice conservative medicine through the end of 1985, savings would total $74,000. My Maxicare bonus for practicing cost-effective, quality medicine would have been $37,000, but this was not to be.

In the fall of 1984, I met a friend from medical school at a Continuing Medical Education (CME) conference in Madison, Wisconsin. Dr. Larry was an Internal Medicine specialist in Green Bay and had been approached by one of his friends regarding a new medical director position being created at Employer's Health Insurance Company (EHIC). EHIC was initiating a managed care product and looking for a medical director; it was the second largest insurer of small employer groups in the country. They sold individual health insurance and coverage to employer groups with fewer than one hundred employees. I knew I was born for this job.

I asked Larry to contact his friend and let him know I was interested in applying for the position. Jack M., the Vice President of the legal department and internal corporate counsel for EHIC, called. We arranged a dinner meeting in February 1985. The meeting went very well. I was invited to interview with the executive management team and tour the company.

The Offer I Could Not Refuse

On a warm spring day in 1985, I left my office early one Friday and drove north on Highway 41 for interviews with the executives of Employer's Health

---

4   Centers for Medicare & Medicaid Services. "National Health Expenditure (NHE) Fact Sheet." Retrieved on January 18, 2011 from http://www.cms.gov/NationalHealthExpendData/25_NHE_Fact_Sheet.asp#TopOfPage.

Insurance Company (EHIC). The company is situated in De Pere, Wisconsin, just south of Green Bay on the east side of the highway. The new glass and sprawling white concrete structure is an impressive site. The building and campus are surrounded by low rolling hills and farmland.

The Vice President of the Law Department met me in the foyer and took me to the executive offices on the third floor for interviews with upper management. The executives just returned from a team-building experience in Canada and were in an exceptionally good mood. The team-building event was more of an Outward Bound experience than a vacation.

These were extremely competent executives. After an hour with the Vice President of Human Resources (HR), I was taken for a tour of the facility. As we left his office, the elevator door opened, and Ron Weyers, one of the founders of the company, walked out, pushing a very large mail cart, carrying cases of Miller beer and Pepsi. Ron was on a mission and invited us to walk along. The company was making special efforts to process a back log of medical claims, and the employees had been working past the usual quitting time for a couple of weeks. Ron knew all the employees by their first names. As we walked through several wings, he asked them how things were going and thanked them for the work they were doing. His next query, "Do you want a Miller or a Pepsi?" The choice between beer and soft drinks seemed weighted toward Miller but this was, after all, Green Bay. It was apparent this was a place where the most important assets were the people. These down-to-earth executives had a genuine appreciation for the value of the folks in their work force. I knew I had to work here.

Following these interviews, I was given an offer I could not refuse. Actually, after negotiation of the salary and benefits I was given an offer that cut my income by 25 percent but presented an opportunity that would change my life. The initial organization of the Medical Management Department reported to Jack, the Vice President of the Legal Department. This made sense because of the state compliance and legal issues involved with the product start-up. Jack had also been the executive doing all the research, ground work and planning for the new managed care insurance product. We agreed on a starting date of July 1, 1985.

My memories of the last six months of clinical practice include several significant medical cases and one personal disappointment. One memorable patient was a woman in her early 60s. She was a Maxicare patient with a treatable cancer. She was referred to one of the general surgeons on my panel who removed the cancer, but lymph node biopsy revealed the cancer had spread. An oncology referral to both Radiotherapy and Internal Medicine was authorized. The care was medically necessary, and she had a quality outcome without any complications. At the time I left practice, this patient was cancer free.

I had no second thoughts about referring this patient to surgery or oncology for high cost medical care. I had not been paid $21 per month to care for this patient. I had been allocated $504,000 to care for my population of patients for the year. I knew proper care for this patient consumed about $50,000, but I also understood I had been allocated enough resources to manage all the primary and specialty care for my population of 900 patients.

During this last year, I cared for a young woman with a devastating disease. She was a mother of three in her early 30s, seen in my office on a Monday for abdominal pain and vomiting. She did not have an acute abdomen requiring immediate surgical intervention. There was no history or evidence of intestinal bleeding. She did have tenderness in her upper abdomen. I sent her to the hospital outpatient department for blood tests with instructions to wait there for the results.

Her blood sugar and serum amylase (a test for the condition of the pancreas) were sky high. I admitted her immediately. Over the next twenty-four hours, she deteriorated rapidly as her pancreas digested itself. I knew she was very ill at the time of admission and arranged emergency consultations with a gastroenterologist and surgeon. She deteriorated further over the next twenty-four hours and, because of elevations in other blood chemistry tests, I arranged emergency nephrology, endocrinology and infectious disease consults. The patient progressed to kidney and liver failure and died on Friday.

Because of her age, an autopsy was performed. No cause for the original pancreatitis or progression to total organ failure was found. Bad things happen to good people and can happen in a blink of an eye. Even if appropriate medical care is delivered, the outcome is never predictable. I cannot remember if this family had insurance, but I hope they did. The week of care that ended in this disaster cost an extraordinary amount of money. If such a disaster happened to an uninsured family today, not only would the family face the loss of their mother, they would also face the prospect of bankruptcy.

During the spring of 1985, I sold the office and practice to an emergency room physician, Dr. Upendra. He was an excellent physician who worked in my office at times when I was out of town attending Continuing Medical Education (CME) seminars. He had married Paula, one of the nurses who worked for a time in my Cudahy office. Paula was the daughter of a Milwaukee firefighter, and our families had been close for many years. My office staff would be staying to work with Dr. Upendra and Paula.

I knew the patients and office staff would be in good hands. I explained the contractual relationship with Maxicare and discussed the principles of managed care, including appropriate use of the specialty referral network with the new owners. Dr. Upendra would be taking over the managed care contract on July 1, 1985. Maxicare would not agree to pay the bonus owed me at the end of six months, stating the contract called for payment at the end of the year (December 31, 1995). Dr. Upendra and I agreed to split any bonus due at the end of 1985. All the loose ends seemed to be tied up, but before I would leave, I would be very disappointed with my staff.

My wife and I had been very fiscally responsible during my clinical practice years. With the help of our accountant, lawyer and stockbroker, retirement accounts had been initiated for the employees and me. Our children's Clifford Trust was substantial and would eventually cover all their higher education needs. The retirement accounts complied with the IRS maximum contribution rules. At the time I left practice, all my employees were fully vested. The individual employee retirement accounts varied from $9,000 to $18,000.

These monies had to be transferred into the employees' individual IRAs when the business changed hands. I talked to the staff about the value these accounts would have at retirement age, especially if they continued to contribute to their funds. I had our stockbroker, who could manage the accounts, make a presentation regarding the future value of this money. At a minimum, the dollars would have doubled every seven years. If the employees added a small amount of money every year, their IRAs could provide a more comfortable retirement.

These were good, intelligent people, but they all cashed out their retirement accounts, paying income tax and early withdrawal penalties to the IRS. I was very disappointed but learned a very important principle. Most people will opt for the short-term gain, regardless of the long-term consequences. This is just human nature and takes great effort and discipline to resist.

This focus on short-term gain regardless of long-term consequences also appears to be the way American business functions. The quarterly report becomes all-important and must show positive numbers or the stock price will drop. Sometimes the long-term consequences are not so long-term. The recent Wall Street financial services crash and our burst housing bubble illustrate this point.

For a few short years of excessive profits making very rich people even richer, the economy of the nation was sacrificed. Their "better angels" never touch many people in their personal lives or business affairs. There has to be a reasonable level of government regulation to protect us from ourselves and from those around us who would do harm.

Kathy and I spent several weeks preparing for the move to Green Bay. I located a furnished rental apartment and moved to Green Bay on July 1. Kathy,

Jill and Mark would stay in Milwaukee until the end of summer and join me before the school year. Our daughter, Jill, and son, Mark, were entering their senior and junior years at South Milwaukee High School, but they adjusted to the new high school in Green Bay in a matter of a few days.

The Employers Health relocation package included the cost of the physical move and living expenses for six months. The home in Milwaukee was sold in a short time. We decided to have a home built in Green Bay. The moving company would store our furniture until our new home was completed. The Human Resource Department of Employers Health facilitated the relocation.

I left clinical practice on June 30 and started my new career in administrative medicine on July 1, 1985. I believed I had been practicing cost-effective, quality medicine and learned a great deal about managed care through some training and significant practical experience. I was about to discover that I knew and understood very little about managed care or insurance. It would take several years for me to discover that I knew essentially nothing at that time about measuring quality care or the process of quality improvement.

I learned my "common sense" approach to medical necessity was not standardized, reproducible or scalable. I believed my style of medical practice demonstrated a high level of care coordination and, considering my education, training and experience, may have been doing so at a level near to the top of my peer group of general and family practitioners. I would learn that effective coordination of care could be carried out at several levels of magnitude higher than where I had been. I believed that my office charts were reasonably well organized, facilitating effective delivery of health care, and that my filing system was efficient. I would learn I was living in a paper storm and usually practicing incident medicine.

I discovered early on that the EHIC folks and I were on a very steep managed care learning curve, and they were not that far ahead of me. They had not hired me to reproduce the workflows I developed in response to the issues of private solo practice. My positive attitude toward managed care and my problem solving capability were the reasons I was hired.

To be effective and successful in this new position, I had to master the administrative side of medicine, managed care and insurance. In effect, this would be on-the-job Master's level business training. I was reminded of my first days at Marquette Medical School. I was looking at a very large mountain of coal and needed to start shoveling.

PART THREE
Health Insurance Administration
1985–2000

Chapter 5:
Administrative Medicine

Ron Weyers and Wally Hilliard founded Wisconsin Employers Group (WEG) in 1969 and sold policies to small groups and individuals. Financial issues in the early 1980s resulted in the sale of WEG to American Express, which also owned Fireman's Fund, for $10 million, and WEG was renamed Employers Health Insurance Company (EHIC). Ron and Wally stayed on board to manage company operations. Fireman's Fund was spun off, but American Express kept EHIC. In the late 1980s, the company would be sold to Lincoln National Insurance (LNC) for $215 million. EHIC became part of LNC's Employee Benefits Division. Within a year of this sale, Ron and Wally would be gone.

So I left fourteen years of private practice on the south side of Milwaukee and entered a full-time administrative career in managed care. During my last five years of practice, I developed and managed South Shore IPA, a small Independent Practice Association. It had been a "gatekeeper" model, where the physicians were given the financial resources and incentives to provide cost effective medical care to members of the health care plan.

The model worked poorly for doctors with practice patterns primarily based on Fee for Service (FFS) reimbursement. The adjustment to a financial system that emphasized population management was impossible for most of the more 130 physicians initially recruited to this program, which had dwindled to a "gang of ten" by the time I left—less than 10 percent were able to comprehend the program goals and adapt their practices and habits. This is likely representative of most doctors across the country. A person paid to plant trees by the sprout does not necessarily make the best forest ranger or resource manager.

Employers Health Insurance Company: 1985 to 1990

I had been hired by EHIC to develop capacity at the company for the care management for the new State of Wisconsin-approved health maintenance plans. I had been brought in because of my problem-solving skills and understanding of the basics of managed care. I had not been hired to bring the gatekeeper HMO model to the company. It took a short adjustment time for me to make this paradigm shift.

The EHIC HMO was a "group model" plan. In this model, EHIC contracted with medium- to large-sized medical group practices to care for plan members. We paid the groups a monthly fee for each assigned member of the plan to cover all primary and specialty services. In return for this monthly capitation fee for each member, the group assumed the financial risk for managing and delivering care to their assigned patient population.

The EHIC plan was not operationally different from the initial gatekeeper model I had been practicing. EHIC did not dictate how the group distributed or allocated their monthly capitation. The contracted medical group determined the reimbursement formula for their individual physicians. Most groups used a formula that included a Fee for Service (FFS) production component.

We expected the doctors to practice cost effective quality medicine and to avoid providing or ordering unnecessary care. Success of this model depended on the abilities of the clinic's medical director and administrative staff to facilitate delivery of quality, cost effective care. The medical director was generally a practicing physician and highly regarded mentor. Other physicians, in consultation regarding appropriate and necessary care plans, could call upon him or her when any issues arose requiring their mentor's advice.

This capitation model generated several unusual and unintended consequences. The clinics were given the monthly per member capitation up front. By contract, the clinics were to report patient interactions to EHIC for financial reporting. In the HMO world, the records of patient interactions with the clinic physicians are called "encounters" rather than "claims" or "bills." These data are for informational and management purposes as no FFS payment checks are processed. Capitation was the means to pre-pay for all primary and specialty clinic services.

EHIC provided financial reports to the clinic administration for presentation to the physicians at their monthly business meetings. These reports would show the physicians and clinic administrators *who was naughty* and *who was nice*. The reports indicated which doctors were practicing cost effective medicine and those who were breaking the bank. Capitation transferred the financial risk for the assigned population to the group and their physicians. The meetings to determine how to split the pie between the doctors must have been very interesting.

Most clinic administrators had difficulty with the paradigm shift from claims submission to secure FFS reimbursement to submission of non-reimbursable encounter data for capitated patients to generate management reports. Submitting encounter data was seen as an administrative burden, not as a management information resource. After all, they had the money up front and believed they knew what to do with it. EHIC needed to process the paper work to generate data to determine where the money was going. These data were needed to price the HMO product appropriately and assure the capitation covered medically necessary services delivered by the contracted clinics. This process ran into early difficulties because the new EHIC information system was not up to the task.

The massive managed care database computer program was called the "Badger" Information System. Medical management decisions were part of the encounter processing and claims adjudication process. Badger was initially only designed to process encounters without printing checks. After more than six months of system redesign and full data integration, the new "Badger" managed care encounter and claims processing system was up and running.

Once operational, Badger produced encounter data and financial reports for the clinic administrators and medical directors. One of my tasks as EHIC medical director was to travel across the State of Wisconsin with a Provider Relations Account Manager to present these reports at clinic meetings. The relationship between EHIC and the partner clinics worked well after the computer systems became aligned and the players understood the managed care principals.

EHIC retained the financial risk for hospitalization and specialty referrals. The written workflow required an authorization by the medical department before these specialty and hospital claims could be adjudicated and checks cut. The EHIC medical department nurses monitored referrals to outside specialists and hospital admissions, but claim payment authorizations for such referrals were usually effectively rubber stamped. Unfortunately, the old claims processing system had no direct link between the claims adjudicator and the medical management nurse. Before the conversion to the new Badger Information System, claim reviewers could approve payment without checking the medical authorization computer screens. This verification was not always done, since the claims processors, like my mother at the cosmetics factory, were piece workers and their performance evaluations depended on the number of claims processed. Quality improvement reports for claims processing accuracy were available to claims managers and supervisors, but when push came to shove and a backlog piled up... well, you get the picture.

Length of Stay Benefit Determination at EHIC

Initial managed care efforts focused on reducing the number of hospital days per thousand insured lives. Excessive length of hospital stays (LOS) was the big problem. Early on, EHIC had neither the administrative medical staff nor the universally accepted medical necessity standards of care to screen physician admission or referral requests. Standards were put into place when EHIC managed care products were marketed. Interqual, a company that published "average" LOS tables, was used to determine an initial LOS authorization for the admission diagnosis. A short time later, EHIC added severity of illness criteria developed by Milliman & Robertson to the authorization process.

The EHIC utilization review nurses never questioned the medical necessity of a physician's hospital admission notification. All requests for hospitalization authorizations were approved. The Interqual LOS tables were used to set a "review date" just short of the average stay. On this prescribed day, the medical necessity of continued in-patient care would be assessed. The idea was to get ahead of the LOS averages to push for the minimum number of medically necessary days.

A nurse in the medical department at EHIC called the floor nurse caring for the patient at the hospital. They would discuss information about the level of care the patient required; the content of these conversations was logged into the comment pages of the Badger Information System. The utilization nurse could authorize payment for additional days if the patient required intensive monitoring, extensive treatment or twenty-four hour nursing care. The medically necessary level of service justified the additional LOS.

The review nurse would suspend (but not deny) payment authorization for extended LOS if the care delivered did not meet the intensity of service screens, or if the insured did not require twenty-four hour nursing care. If the EHIC nurse could not establish the medical necessity of continued hospital care, and the attending physician did not write the discharge order, she referred the case to me. Nurses never themselves denied authorization of payment for care; medical director action was required if the review nurse found that the patient's condition, as documented by the PCP, failed to meet medical criteria to justify payment authorization for the requested service or test. I would call the attending physician to discuss the most appropriate place of service (POS) for the intended plan of treatment. During fifteen years of administration as an HMO medical director, I never told a physician that a patient must be discharged. I informed many physicians that payment for additional LOS would terminate when additional in-patient days did not meet medical necessity criteria.

The process was very straightforward. The attending doctor determined the plan of treatment. Universally accepted standards were available to determine the most appropriate and cost effective place for delivery of medical services ordered by the physician. Reimbursement authorization for ongoing in-patient care was determined based on the appropriateness of place of service. During the early days of managed care, medical directors rarely discussed the appropriateness of the care with the attending physician. In spite of very loose reigns, the medical department significantly reduced the number of in-patient days per thousand HMO members. We were getting doctors to think about what they were doing, and we were getting the statistics together to show what effective care could mean.

"Practicing" Medicine verses "Administering" Medicine

It is very important at this point to understand the difference between "authorizing payment" and "ordering medical care." Only the licensed physician may practice medicine. The practice of medicine is defined in state law and regulations. Only the licensed physician may order or deliver care to the patient. The insurance company, government bureaucrat, administrator and medical director are not licensed to provide care, order care or deny care.

The state government defines and regulates the practice of medicine and the business of financing medical care. The state board of medical examiners defines and regulates the practice of medicine including licensing of physicians. The state insurance commissioner defines and regulates the business of insurance including all interactions between the insurance company and the public. These regulatory bodies are separate and distinct stovepipes of state government.

State regulators approve all insurance company and HMO documents. Health care plan language, benefit design and premiums are regulated by the state. No insurance company document is made public or used for marketing without approval of a state bureaucrat. The matching of the medical services delivered, with the language defining covered benefits, must be precise and consistent. Failure to do so for the process of approval or denial invites unfair claims practice litigation.

The practicing physician has a duty to her patient to provide quality medical care and services. The duty of the medical director, working at any fiscal intermediary (insurance company or HMO), is to determine if the care ordered or delivered is a covered benefit as defined in the patient's health care plan. The HMO medical director is an interpreter or translator between the patient's medical record as documented by the practicing physician and the contractual language of the insurance or HMO plan.

Inconsistent benefit authorization or denial determinations result in arbitrary and capricious decisions. Some have lead to multimillion-dollar judgments for unfair claims practices. This was one of the major reasons the Badger System had to directly link the medical department authorization with claims payment. Arbitrary payment decisions by claims processors or their supervisors were eliminated. All I had to worry about were arbitrary decisions made by my staff or me.

After fourteen years in primary care practice, including five years of organizing and administering a gatekeeper model IPA, I understood the difference between *practicing* medicine and *administering* a contract. I had not been hired by EHIC to consult with physicians regarding "proper quality care" for their patients. My purpose was to administer the health care contract and develop the Medical Management Department. EHIC valued my knowledge of medicine regarding application of customers' medical information, as presented by the practicing physician, to the insurance business functions of underwriting and proper claims administration.

Over the years, I would discover that many folks working in the insurance industry— most physicians, virtually all patients and all politicians—fail to understand this distinction. This concept is one of the foundation blocks of managed care that crumbled under the weight of popular misconception and political pressure in the later 1990s. The medical-industrial complex won battles while the American public was losing the war for quality, cost effective care.

Tuesday, January 28, 1986 at 12:39 p.m., Central Standard Time, the space shuttle Challenger blew up 73 seconds into the launch. The Shuttle crew included Christa McAuliffe, the first teacher in the space program. Due to the publicity and hype surrounding this launch, many adults and most schoolchildren were watching as the shuttle blasted off.

A group of us watched television in one of the conference rooms. We were stunned. The disaster was investigated for several months. The Rogers Commission found that NASA's organizational culture and decision-making processes had been the key contributing factors to the accident. Financial considerations, ignorance and flawed decision-making by the managers on the ground had resulted in the death of seven people.

This sounded too much like the American medical care system for my comfort. At least in the aviation industry, the pilot is·in the plane with the passengers. As a result, the pilot is very conscientious about performing the pre-flight checklist. American physicians seldom use medical checklists.

Perhaps this is because a catastrophic medical decision failure by a physician results only in the death of the patient.

Behind the Scenes as EHIC Medical Director: The Importance of the Underwriter

Shortly after I started work at EHIC, my duties as the Vice President of Medical Affairs took shape and my calendar began to fill. My primary responsibilities included directing the Medical Management Department personnel and making the final determination to authorize or deny health care plan benefits for those cases failing to meet medical necessity criteria. I was also responsible for development of departmental policies and procedures. In addition, I worked with the Provider Relations Department, independent agents and advised underwriters. On occasion, I traveled with a provider relations representative or insurance agent to explain our medical management policies and procedures to our physician partners or employer clients. My work with the Underwriting Department was more structured and regularly scheduled. The underwriters wanted input from a medical expert with a crystal ball to advise them regarding the rating or possible denial of individual insurance policy applications. Ultimately, the buck stopped at my desk and it was all about cost-effective medical care, customer satisfaction and business retention.

I had a glass-walled office in the executive wing. The newly created Medical Department consisted of a manager, Virginia Yunker, R.N., and three nurses. These folks originally reported to the Claims Department where the nurses had been responsible for retrospective review of medical records for special, high cost claims. If they identified possible abuse, fraud or covered-up preexisting conditions, the case would be referred to an outside physician consultant. I assumed the responsibility to review these cases with the nurses and make recommendations regarding action to our legal department. The focus of the department would change from retrospective (after-the-fact review), to prospective (preauthorization for care) determination of benefits based on compliance with medical standards and criteria. The nurses were ecstatic to be part of the new Medical Management Department and functioning as medical managers. By the time of my departure four years later, the department numbered ninety-one medical professionals.

I shared an administrative assistant with the Vice President of Marketing. This close working relationship resulted in a deeper understanding of insurance marketing and sales. The Marketing Department developed health plan brochures and other sales materials that the Wisconsin Department of Insurance needed to approve prior to printing. Regulatory compliance was especially important for marketing materials. The Marketing Department also managed communication with the independent agents.

To stay competitive and profitable, EHIC placed great emphasis on customer satisfaction and business retention. Our customers were: 1) the insured patients, 2) their employers and 3) independent insurance agents. The insurance agents were the central player in the business model. They needed an innovative product (the insurance plans) to sell and competitive compensation for their sales efforts. I worked with several of our most productive independent agents explaining our medical management programs during sales presentations to larger employers. Our marketing and sales efforts were quite successful: although group contracts are renewed on a yearly basis, EHIC kept a client employer in a unique insurance plan for about three years.

State-licensed independent insurance agents sold the majority of EHIC insurance plans. EHIC paid their state license fee. The marketing department developed new health plan designs and constantly adjusted commission and bonus programs to buy the loyalty of the independent agent sales force. EHIC paid agents a substantial commission based on the premium dollar for the insurance policies these agents sold. The profitability of the insurance agent's book of cases was tracked over the one-year contract period. EHIC paid large bonuses for recruiting new business and retaining profitable accounts.

The agents were the connection between the small business owner and the Underwriting Department. Underwriters are at the heart of the risk management process. They offer the best educated guess about how much it will cost to provide medical care to a group of individuals. This determines the projected overall cost of the benefits plan. The projected medical cost plus administration determines the premium offered to employers for coverage of their employees. Close working relationships existed between the agents and the underwriters, who were skillful at predicting the yearly medical costs for the employer groups evaluated.

I was assigned a second smaller office in the Underwriting Department, where I spent two afternoons a week discussing risk management with the underwriters. One of my duties was to provide input regarding potential medical losses for their more difficult cases. The underwriters were the entry point for new business. They were responsible for determining adjustments to the standard premium for both new and repeat business. The underwriter was responsible for making the business decision to accept, up-rate or deny the application for medical coverage. My role was only advisory.

EHIC tracked the underwriters' book of business to determine their actual individual medical loss ratio. Their supervisors reviewed this information for process improvement and performance review. EHIC also tracked the production and loss ratios of independent agents, so we could properly reward the high producers of profitable businesses.

The underwriters generally had a great deal of latitude in making rating decisions. I would meet with three to five underwriters twice a week. They would have a list of complicated new business and group renewal medical problems to discuss. One such case was from a small group applying for renewal of coverage for their fourteen employees and twenty-seven dependents. A mix of individual coverage and family plans was involved.

The employer experienced a significant medical loss due to the cost of a cardiac revascularization procedure for one of the dependents. This company had been part of the underwriter's book of business for several years, and their loss ratio had always been as projected. This employee's heart surgery had been an unforeseen event and was not part of a known pre-existing condition. The business owner and independent agent were tight and the agent and underwriter were tight. No one involved wanted this business placed with another insurance company.

I reviewed the medical information. The insured suffered an acute event that resulted in very expensive cardiac surgery. The surgery had been a success and recovery unremarkable, with all cardiac parameters returning to normal. We needed to answer several questions before the underwriters could make a determination. Should the employer policy be denied renewal or continued? If renewed, should the premium be rated up, and if so, by how much?

During the renewal process, an underwriter cannot add a pre-existing exclusion to a policy, and it would not be ethical to do so. The medical expense loss for the prior contract year was *water over the dam*. Looking forward, the medical loss would only increase slightly by the cost of a few specialty visits. I advised the underwriter to renew the coverage, with a very small increase in premium, to cover the minor expected additional cost. The underwriter, with my medical input, made a proper justifiable decision, and all involved were satisfied with the outcome, especially the employer and the agent.

Evaluating renewals was relatively uncomplicated compared to evaluating potential new business. EHIC needed at least a year of claim history to determine a fair, justifiable action about a group renewal. New business did not have any past history to help make these determinations and could present a special management risk.

For example, the underwriter would not have to think twice about an application from an employer with five workers, two of whom have brittle diabetes (e.g., poorly controlled diabetes where the patient experiences wild swings in blood sugar), a condition that will be very costly to the insurance company every year. A field agent with any common sense would not even submit such a case. As long as access to health care financing is through employment, this small employer group is essentially uninsurable. The risk of expensive medical complications is just too great. The financial risk to either a for-profit or a not-for-profit insurance company for such a small employer group is unmanageable.

Larger employers provide more flexibility to the underwriter. For example, a group of thirty-five healthy employees and one employee with recent colon cancer surgery might be insurable. If the group policy were written to exclude pre-existing diseases of the colon, specifically for colon cancer, this one individual would not get coverage for the condition but could have coverage for routine visits and other medical necessities, and full coverage could be offered to the rest of the group. The individual with the pre-existing exclusion for colon disease would have coverage for all other conditions within the terms and limitations of the contract. Without the option of pre-existing condition exclusion, the premium for the group could be unaffordable or the entire group might be rejected.

The length or term of the contract affects both the underwriting process and the benefit structure. Buying medical insurance is not like getting married. It is not, "until death do us part." Most employers purchasing health care insurance understand the value of a generous plan with great service, and are willing to pay for quality… up to a point. After all, in the small employer market, the owner was purchasing coverage for his/her family, as well as for the employees. Business owners therefore have a very personal incentive to get the best plan possible for the most reasonable rates—the health care of their own families is at stake. Employers find it is prudent to shop around and seek the best health care plan they can afford at each contract renewal. Competition in the marketplace results in significant turnover pressure for most insurance companies.

Health insurance is a short-term game for this reason. The structure of our health care financing system discourages the long view. The Marketing, Sales and Underwriting Departments were not concerned about the medical loss ratio ten years out, they were only worried about profit in the projected year. Any preventive health care benefit represented increased short-term medical loss, with no short-term financial or medical benefit. A non-smoker with a health club membership had little value in this environment. Wellness programs added short term cost with virtually no short term benefit to the insurance company.

Understanding financial risk management is the key to understanding the current dysfunctional health care system. The yearly insurance contract spreads the financial risk of the individual to a pool of participants through their employer to the insurance company for a negotiated monthly premium. Underwriting small employer group and individual health insurance policies is used to manage the great risk the insurance company takes on when all administrative and health care costs are "owned" for the term of the insurance contract.

Underwriting, at its core, is an educated guess about the projected medical costs for a self-employed individual or small group of employed individuals. Underwriting, and the techniques used by underwriters to assure profitability, will continue as long as Americans access health care financing through employment in relatively small numbers. From the largest employers of thousands to small business owners this system spreads great risk across small populations, thus increasing costs to everyone, regardless of which type of health insurance plan the employer chooses to offer.

The logical alternative to this dysfunctional system is to disconnect health care financing from its access through employment. Employers and self-employed individuals would eliminate insurance premiums and substitute a smaller community rate withholding tax. Private insurance companies would continue to offer Medicare programs and compete as they do now, but these competitive health care plans would be available to everyone. When all taxpayers cover every American, all Americans will become part of the largest self-insured, self funded group in the world. The financial risk for all covered medical goods and services is then spread universally across all taxpayers. The Medicare Metropolitan Service Area health care cost would index the local "community rate" to determine the individual worker withholding tax by geographical area.

There would be no need for underwriting universal health insurance because all individuals in the US would be the population base; healthy individuals who cost the system very little will in effect balance the costs of those with expensive diseases. The underwriting concepts of limitations, pre-existing condition exclusions, variable rating/premium, rescission and cancellation become meaningless. Additionally, universal health insurance is universally portable; it goes with the individual and can be taken from job to job, from employment to self-employment to unemployment, with no lapses in benefits through any transition. This is an important point. According to US Bureau of Labor Statistics, individuals average about 11 jobs during their working years, and 94 percent leave each job before they reach the five-year mark with any given employer.[5] This kind of turnover in Americans' working

---

5   US Bureau of Labor Statistics. (2010, September 10). Economic News Release: "Number of Jobs Held, Labor Market Activity, and Earnings Growth Among the Youngest Baby Boomers: Results From a Longitudinal Survey Summary." Retrieved on December 27, 2010 from http://www.bls.gov/news.rclcase/nlsoy.nr0.htm.

lives is very disruptive to the possibility of managing their health or the potential for continuity of care with in-network providers. Universal health insurance eliminates this problem. By gaining this control of their health care financing, Americans will be better able to manage their own health with the providers they have come to trust, regardless of their employment.

Quality Improvement Training

EHIC sent me to Pennsylvania for medical director training with US Health Care. US Health Care was a "member organization," not an insurance company. They operated "staff model" HMOs, which are operationally similar to the military and one of the prototypical health maintenance organizations, Kaiser Permanente. Physicians working in a classical staff model HMO are salaried rather than reimbursed using a fee for service (FFS) payment schedule. During the two-week training period, my eyes were opened wide through observing the operations in various facilities. Especially impressive was a patient care meeting attended by all the specialists involved in the treatment of several cancer patients. This was similar to but much more productive than the grand rounds I attended at Marquette Medical School.

The primary care provider (PCP), an internist caring for the patient, would present the case. The radiologist presented the imaging studies and explained the findings. The pathologist, using a projection microscope, showed the biopsy slides and explained the cellular abnormalities. The oncologist delineated the disease process and presented the therapeutic alternatives, based on the latest recommendations from peer-reviewed medical journals. The pharmacist discussed possible interactions and complications of potential drug therapies. The team discussed alternative plans of treatment. The group reached a consensus about the most appropriate treatment options.

When the physicians finished discussing the case, the patient and family entered the conference room. The team presented possible options for therapy to the patient and family. The PCP explained the recommended treatment plan, possible complications, and outcome expectations to the patient and family in lay terms. The PCP or the appropriate specialist answered questions from the patient and family members. All members of the team, the doctors and the family members, agreed on the best option.

Until that day, I did not understand what managed care was really about. I had no idea about the level of quality care a multispecialty team of HMO physicians could deliver. The two weeks I spent in training at US Health Care were brilliantly enlightening. This experience affirmed that my choice of a new career in managed care was right.

The owners of EHIC were believers in Continuous Quality Improvement

(CQI). Upper management did not simply say the employees were the company's most important asset, they believed in the concept and managed accordingly. They walked the talk. The corporation paid for extensive training and education in CQI. Everyone had a copy of Out of the *Crisis*[6] by Dr. W. Edwards Deming and Deming Management *Method*[7] by Mary Walton and Dr. Deming. Managers understood that they were not there to filter information coming from the executives. They were there to mentor employees and to help them get the job done and done well—they were there to do the thing right and do the right thing.

Departments in any organization may be viewed as "stove pipes," each with its own chain of command. A major element of the corporate culture at EHIC was the implementation of Deming Point Nine, the removal of barriers between departments. The opinions and suggestions for improvement from employees were highly valued. Employees who submitted ideas for improvement that were put in place were given a small monetary bonus called a "Spot Award." These were good times.

The executives were students of sound business practices and made them operational. A core group of executives attended a W. Edwards Deming quality improvement seminar, where the great man gave a lecture. Dr. Deming has a lot to do with the reason many Americans drive Japanese cars as his principles and Fourteen Points[8] were first adopted by those manufacturing giants.

I could see where quality improvement business principles had direct application to the practice of medicine and how his Seven Deadly Diseases of Western Management[9] have application to both medicine and business. Although Deming had not specifically addressed how to apply his fourteen principals of Total Quality Management (TQM) to the medical delivery system, he did recognize "Excessive Medical Costs" as one of the deadly diseases destroying American businesses. Those seven are: 1) inconsistent purpose; 2) emphasis on the short term; 3) management by fear; 4) unwarranted mobility of top management; 5) over reliance on "known" factors when many are unknown; 6) EXCESSIVE MEDICAL COSTS; and 7) excessive legal damages based on lawyers' contingency fees. If the American economy is to survive, we must certainly address the Deadly Diseases identified by Dr. Deming.

---

6   W. Edwards Deming. (1986). *Out of the Crisis.* Cambridge, MA: MIT Press.

7   Mary Walton and W. Edwards Deming, (1986). *The Deming Management Method.* NY: The Berkley Publishing Group.

8   See Appendix.

9   See Appendix.

The Financial Crash of 1987

On Black Monday, October 19, 1987, the Stock Market dropped over 20 percent (over 500 points) resulting in what my stockbroker called "a paper loss." He meant nothing would be lost if we did not panic and sell our stocks—selling low when the economy has time to recover is a recipe for individual disaster and a longer crash. We preferred Bailey frugality to Potter's pennies on the dollar.[10] Retirement was a long way off for us, so the value of our retirement portfolio had time to recover. The employees who bailed out of their retirement plans when I left practice probably thought they had made a good decision. It was my belief they made the wrong move. There was no reason to panic. After all, this particular downturn did prove to be just a paper loss for those who stuck it out. I was working and would be for a long time. I knew the market would come back, and my retirement account would recover.

In late spring of 1988, Dr. Norm Schroeder began work as my Assistant Medical Director. Norm was cajoled into starting just before May 31 to get the full 1000 hours for the year and qualify for the 401K retirement plan. EHIC structured this retirement program open to all employees. Valuing employees was not just a slogan; it was part of the corporate culture that embodied the Deming philosophy. The company matched contributions made by the worker, up to the limit of the IRS regulations. I contributed the maximum allowed executives. Norm followed my advice and did the same. My ongoing contributions would come into the retirement account at the bottom of the market and grow substantially (buying low, the best way to enter the market).

I thought Ronny and the Republicans would surely fix the economy. It was their top priority, since they, and the rest of the movers and shakers at the top of the economic food chain, had a lot more to lose than the rest of us. I was convinced that trickle-down economics should help bring the economy back and besides, being in the middle of the economic food chain, I was one of the people doing some of the trickling. My position and salary were secure, so there was no need to wait for the trickle from above. Tax cuts for the wealthy

---

10 In "It's a Wonderful Life," during the 1929 stock market crash George Bailey convinces enough of the Building and Loan customers to keep their savings in his institution rather than lose half of their investment from selling their shares to Mr. Potter's rival bank. This saves his customers from potentially facing much greater long-term losses, and saves the Building and Loan from closing through a run on the bank. (Capra, Frank (Producer & Director). (1947). *It's a Wonderful Life* (Motion Picture). USA: Liberty Films II).

and a reduction of the social services budget did the trick, and the economy improved... for a while.

Except for the Iran-Contra affair and the World Court finding America guilty of war crimes against Nicaragua, the country believed Ronny and the Republicans governed well. The economy responded positively. We had not yet experienced the serious downturn resulting from *Reaganomics* and the policies of "supply-side economics."

By the 1988 election, the economy was doing reasonably well, and during his campaign, Vice President George H. W. Bush promised, "No new taxes." The image of Dukakis' bobble head sticking out of a hatch of a tank still comes to mind. The presidential campaign between George H. W. Bush and Michael Dukakis during 1988 was another walk in the park for Republicans. I voted for George the First.

EHIC Community Involvement

During my first several years at EHIC, I volunteered at the local Green Bay Free Clinic, seeing patients several mornings per month. I also volunteered as a ringside physician for a VFW post that held boxing matches between local clubs and those from the Milwaukee area. I enjoyed seeing patients and felt a need *to keep one foot* in the practice of medicine. I was wrong to think this minimal patient contact would provide me with some degree of credibility with our network practicing physicians.

Employers Health Insurance Company (EHIC) supported the Clinic when the economy was good. During construction of the new building, I secured funding for a second hard wire connection system in the walls. The contractor installed the hard wires (at very low cost) before covering the free clinic walls with sheet rock. This network of wires connected the telephone switching room with each examination room desk.

The hard wiring was in preparation for the secure computerized medical record system I could see on the horizon. I believed the Clinic would make an excellent test site for directly connecting a local medical practice computer system with the main claim processing software system at EHIC. When completely developed, such a system could be scaled up and migrated to our partner clinics, eliminating paper submission, data entry errors, rework and delays. Electronic fund transfer in a matter of seconds could return payment for services covered by the benefit plans.

The company hired consultants to write a massive database computer program ("Badger") for administering the HMO products and processing claims. We planned to link the new Badger System to an electronic medical record and billing system at the free clinic using a dedicated telephone line.

The hard-wired configuration offered significant security over the wireless technology now available. However, as the economy declined, so did financial support for the clinic computer system. The installation did not happen during my time with EHIC.

Utilization Review and Case Management at EHIC

During the second half of the 1980s, care was "managed" through the processes of "Utilization Review" (UR) and "Case Management" (CM) using medical criteria and standards of care. Committees of physicians from the public and private sectors spent many years developing these standards. Managed care organizations (MCOs) applied these medical standards and criteria to evaluate the information presented by the practicing physician during the UR process. Matching the documented patient information with the standards of care and the insurance contract resulted in authorization or denial of the requested benefit.

The process of case management (CM), under the direction of the patient's primary care provider (PCP), helped navigate the complexities of our medical-industrial complex to maximize effective use of available benefits. A CM nurse assisted with the physician's management of a group of insured patients. These patients corresponded to the nurse's area of interest and expertise. For example, one of our nurses would be assigned patients with global head injuries. Another might manage the benefits for infants in neonatal intensive care units.

The CM process worked almost like a buyers' club, where the nurse was the professional shopping assistant. The physician would be the fashion consultant and the patient the customer. The customer is free to shop anywhere if paying out of pocket, but following the shopping assistant's guidance will help the customer (patient) save money. The idea is to execute the fashion consultant's recommended look (treatment plan for whatever ails the patient), using buyer's club outlets (approved medical facilities and specialists), to stretch the available dollars. The goal is to underwrite quality care within the terms and limitations of the contract.

The health care plan is a contract between the employer, the risk managing claims administrator (the insurance company) and the employee. One of the central concepts in contract law is, "If it is not written, it does not exist." That is about all I understand regarding contract law. Many medical professionals do not understand this much.

Several years into development of the EHIC medical management capability, a problem developed in Case Management. One of the nurse managers did not understand the difference between maximizing the benefits of the plan and inventing new benefits not included in the plan. On several occasions, she extended a limited benefit, or authorized an excluded service, by reducing or eliminating a different defined benefit. The transition from caring for patients in a clinical setting to administering a benefit plan for insured patients in a business environment was very difficult for most medical professionals, and impossible for some.

For example, some group contracts limit payment for both the number of in-facility rehabilitation days, and out-patient rehabilitation visits. The nurse could not create coverage for additional out-patient services by using existing facility in-patient days (called an "*in-lieu-of*" exchange). By contract, the number of in-facility days provided cannot be taken away or altered by an arbitrary decision of a nurse manager. If, at some point in the future, the insured required re-admission to the facility and the nurse denied the benefit for the re-admission (the days having been "used up" in the arbitrary *in-lieu-of* decision) EHIC could be accused of unfair claims practices. In addition, there was no way to standardize how many *in-lieu-of* days each case manager would switch around. Arbitrary decisions about how many days over the limit that the benefit plan authorized would also create an unfair claims practice liability. These arbitrary decisions were not the solution to what was obviously a problem for some patients.

Eight years and several employers later, I would solve the benefit conundrum through my use of contract language. Case Managers, with medical director approval, were allowed to authorize a monthly case management global fee for specific disease states (e.g., diabetes and asthma). It was then up to the medical providers to determine how to use the available global fee to reach a quality outcome for their patients.

State Compliance at EHIC

In these early days, state insurance regulators monitored the legislated quality assurance (QA) requirements. The EHIC compliance officer reported to the Vice President of the Law Department, and was part of our internal checks and balances. The state performed site visits yearly to determine if the HMO was in compliance with all insurance regulations, and especially those concerning utilization review (UR), case management (CM) and QA.

With the rigorous day-to-day business responsibilities, state compliance requirements were usually on a back burner. Most of the executives did not look forward to a visit from our compliance officer. Some corporate officers functioned like physicians that are never able to keep up with required hospital paperwork. The compliance officer was a very special person who was able to push for compliance gently. Everyone understood she had the backing of the Senior Vice President of the Legal Department so she never had to push too hard.

The Medical Department Quality Assurance Program (QA Program) was a medical management tool and a state regulation requirement. Compliance with the QA Program was more difficult than regulatory requirements for UR and CM for which the credentials, tools and criteria used were established, standardized and easily documented. During these early days, no cookbook existed for meeting state QA compliance requirements. There was more art and nuance than basic science involved in satisfying the state reviewers.

The medical management department had little difficulty meeting state reviewer standards because we understood quality improvement after our training in Deming quality improvement philosophy and techniques. I developed and managed the HMO Quality Assurance Program. Within this program, three network-wide quality-of-care studies were designed, directed and completed. These studies enabled the plan to meet all state requirements.

A significant percentage of EHIC's book of business was in the HMO product. The department grew as we hired several nurse managers to manage the increasing workload. The medical department expanded to meet the number of calls asking for benefit pre-certification for selected out-patient services, elective hospital admissions and non-urgent specialist referrals. No managed care organization has ever required pre-authorization of emergency and urgent care. The UR nurses reviewed medical information and claims for these services after the fact.

The UR department used universally accepted criteria and medical standards to establish the medical necessity of the top thirty high cost out-patient procedures. Using the science of clinical epidemiology, the medical community and specialty organizations established the surgical standards and criteria we used. EHIC determined which high cost, frequently abused medical services to review, such as hysterectomy (removing the uterus) and cholecystectomy (removing the gallbladder). Norm and I verified payment of yearly subscriber fees for the criteria manuals used to make the length of stay and benefit decisions. We used these sound, scientifically-based criteria to authorize benefits for such out-patient procedures as CT scans. The criteria determined the medical necessity and benefit determination for admissions for surgical procedures.

The patient and physician determined the treatment plan, but EHIC determined if benefit payment was justified.

The UR nurses reviewed elective hospital admission requests to determine if the physician's treatment plan met medical necessity criteria and met intensity of service criteria justifying hospital admission. For example, if a surgeon requested preauthorization of benefits for a patient's hysterectomy, the medical facts would either justify the procedure or establish that the procedure was not medically necessary. If justified, benefit payment for the procedure and hospitalization were authorized. In other words, if the universally accepted medical criteria confirmed the medical necessity, the benefit payment was authorized.

If the nurse determined the treatment was not justified, the UR nurse referred the case to Norm or me for benefit determination. If we verified the medical facts failed to meet criteria, the benefit for the unnecessary procedure and the associated hospital days were denied. If criteria were not met, the physician making the request had the pleasure of talking to Norm or me. More times than not, extenuating circumstances or errors of omission in the patient medical record were found, and the benefit was authorized. If we could establish, with confidence, that the criteria had not been met, the authorization for benefit payment would be denied.

It is important to understand that Norm and I were denying *payment*, not denying *care*. Only the physician, with consent of the patient, determines what care is *delivered*. Norm and I, as Medical Directors, using universally accepted medical standards and criteria, determined what health care would be *reimbursed*. We authorized or denied payment. We did not practice medicine, or direct the care of any insured patient.

Experimental Exclusion—the Hard Way

This process worked well to determine the medical necessity for payment authorization, where universally accepted standards were available. When it came to making benefit decisions for very complex and possibly experimental procedures, medical care standards and criteria were not as well defined. Norm and I, with input from the legal department, developed a methodology for assessing requests to determine if benefits should be authorized and claims paid, for these complex, and possibly experimental cases.

The Health Care Plan obligated EHIC to pay for medically necessary medical care within the terms and limitations of the contract. The contract excluded benefit payment for experimental procedures. These contract limitations and exclusions had been used to analyze the expected medical costs and to price the Health Care Plan. These financial determinations were based on ballpark industry assumptions about the effectiveness of medical management techniques. The ability of EHIC to remain solvent and meet claim payment obligations of the HMO product depended on proper administration of the benefits.

Services that were covered by contract and determined to be medically necessary had to be paid within the terms and limitations specified. Payment for services that were excluded had to be denied. Any benefit approval request for care that fell into "gray" areas of either medical criteria or contract language had to be paid. For the authorization to be denied, the benefit payment request had to violate specific medical necessity criteria or precisely fit benefit plan limitations and exclusions. If the denial could not be absolutely justified, based on the facts, the request for benefit approval had to be authorized.

If arbitrary and capricious medical necessity and denial decisions were made, EHIC would be open to unfair claims practice litigation. These are the judgments you hear about that come in at tens of millions of dollars, since there is no Employee Retirement Income Security Act (ERISA) protection from such a tort (law suit). Norm and I had to be certain the medical facts, and the process used to make benefit determinations for these special cases were standardized and defensible in court.

If an authorization request to approve benefits for an unusually high-cost treatment was made, medical necessity had to be determined. The medical records of the insured from all treating physicians would be obtained. We would do a literature search to determine if the procedure was the "standard of care." A decision could usually be made after this literature search, but since we were determining benefits, not directing care, an outside benefit consultation would be conducted.

If the literature search seemed to indicate the requested care was experimental, a more intensive evaluation was needed. The patient's medical records would be redacted, removing any information identifying the patient or treating physician. A packet containing the sanitized records and the literature search would be sent, via certified overnight mail, to a practicing medical expert in the appropriate medical specialty. The response would be returned in writing, with a discussion of the requested therapy, and the opinion of the consultant regarding medical necessity and experimental status. Norm or I would consider this additional information when making the benefit authorization decision.

A reasonable man might conclude that this medical benefit determination procedure, for a special high-cost case, would be more than adequate to make a fair, legally defensible payment determination. A reasonable man would be wrong. I was about to learn more than I wanted to know about the difference between medical determinations and the determinations made by administrative judges. The experience would greatly expand my knowledge about experimental medicine and, in the end, simplify benefit determinations. It was a stressful and costly education.

Late in 1988, EHIC received a request for authorization for high dose chemotherapy and autologous bone marrow transplant (ABMT) for treatment of breast cancer. Chemotherapy drugs are poisons that kill cells. They are designed to kill fast growing, rapidly multiplying, cancer cells, while having less effect on stable cells (nerves), and slower reproducing cells (bone marrow, gut lining and hair). The oncologist practices the medical art of poisoning the patient, just enough to kill the cancer cells, while only making the other cells temporarily very sick. If the bone marrow is killed, the patient dies of anemia (no red cells) or infection (no white cells). If the intestines are damaged, the patient dies of dehydration (like having cholera) or infection when bacteria cannot be kept out of the blood. If the patient is kept alive long enough for the weakened cells to recover, the bald patient survives. If the patient survives and all the cancer cells are killed, the patient is cured. Well, at least the five-year survival rate is very high.

One of the critical limits to the amount of poison the patient will live through is the amount of drugs the bone marrow will tolerate. Some cancers require higher levels of poisons than the rest of the cells in the body can survive. If the patient's own bone marrow is sucked out and stored for later reinfusion (an "autologous" infusion), much higher levels of poison can be achieved. Then the gut lining survival becomes the critical limiting factor for how much chemical poison may be administered. High dose chemotherapy is given with the hope the cancer cells are all killed. Of course, all the bone marrow cells and most of the cells lining the gut are also killed. Following chemotherapy, the patient's stored "autologous" bone marrow cells are transfused back into the patient.

This scenario was being tested experimentally in the late 1980s. This human experiment was classified as a Phase I protocol designed to determine the toxicity levels of the chemicals being used. Human experiments are never considered standard care or attempts at cure. If the patient survives the chemo long enough for the transfused marrow cells to take hold, the patient survives. How long the patient would survive was under study.

The insured in this particular case was a young woman diagnosed with advanced breast cancer by her physician. The physician, knowing standard chemotherapy and radiation therapy for this disease was usually not effective, requested referral authorization for his patient to the University of Nebraska Medical Center. The physician referred the patient for human experimentation because he believed no other therapy would be effective.

Following the request and receipt of the medical records by facsimile, the literature search was completed by the next day. Review of the medical information revealed that standard therapy was available and review of contracted specialists in western Wisconsin where the patient lived established that standard care was accessible. The literature also supported the conclusion that the requested therapy at the University of Nebraska Medical Center was an experimental study.

A practicing medical oncologist and professor on the clinical staff of the University of Wisconsin Medical School was called for an opinion regarding the status of the proposed therapy. The outside consultant confirmed the treatment was not available in Wisconsin and was only being performed at three American university medical centers under experimental conditions. One of these sites was the University of Nebraska Medical Center.

Our consultant was told he would receive the documents we assembled for his written report. We would provide the attending PCP a timely verbal denial based on the benefit exclusion. This was done within 48 hours of the request. I believed we connected all the dots between the patient's condition, the practicing physician's authorization request, the status of available therapies and the benefit language in the contract.

Given the state of the art in managed care at the time, our decision-making process and turnaround time were excellent. All the medical facts regarding the case had been identified and evaluated. An outside expert had been consulted and confirmed our determination that the proposed therapy was experimental. The contract language excluding experimental treatment was clear and explicit. The decision was reasoned, fair and timely. What could go wrong?

The insured was the daughter of the owner of one of our larger companies in western Wisconsin. His lawyer contacted our legal department several days after our decision to deny coverage for the experimental therapy was communicated. It was clear our benefit determination would be going to court. This would be an administrative hearing before a judge to determine if the decision of the EHIC medical department should be reversed.

The Employee Retirement Income Security Act (ERISA) became law in 1974 (Pub.L. 93-406, 88 Stat. 829) and protected employee benefits from punitive damage judgments. Protection of health insurance companies by this act may have been an unintended consequence, but there it was. Health care insurance is an employee benefit and immune from punitive damage awards. What was being placed on the table, or rather the judge's bench, was the validity of the decision to deny and if reversed, the cost, within other terms and limitations, of the care in question.

Norm and I met with the Legal Department staff lawyers frequently for the following several weeks. The legal department staff felt the decision process was appropriate. All elements of fact and procedures used to make the decision had to be examined prior to the court appearance to assure the file would be complete. We had a very short time to prepare. The judge fast-tracked the case so if our decision were reversed, therapy would not be unreasonably delayed. This was a reasonable stipulation.

The facts of the case were not in dispute, nor the explicit language excluding experimental medical care. We determined that the case would come down to the literature and our outside expert determining the care was "experimental" vs. the primary care physician determination that the care was "necessary." The central issue became the meaning of the word "experimental." The additional information uncovered through meticulous research about this general topic was very esoteric.

The contract defined "experimental" as treatment that was not considered the "generally accepted practice in the community." This definition triggered several questions: Is it sufficient to define "experimental" in terms of negatives? Is it possible a treatment that is not the community standard will not be experimental? Could a treatment that is not widely available be accepted as standard care?

Expert opinion is just an opinion and not necessarily fact. The literature and our consulting expert supported our benefit determination but would it be enough? A site visit to the University of Nebraska Medical Center was productive, but no additional medical information about the insured was available. The transplant team had not evaluated the patient.

It became clear early on that our day in court was going to be about how the judge could justify compelling EHIC to pay for the experimental procedure. In the end he chose, like Admiral Nelson, to turn a blind eye to the medical facts and base the decision on a disagreement between "experts." The record showed the attending physician considered the care necessary and the consultant, who had not examined the patient, considered the care experimental.

The money EHIC spent to visit the Medical Center, defend the case, and cover the benefit was well worth the price. We gained a great deal of knowledge about how to make experimental determinations and initiated a relationship with a quality transplant center. We were able to modify our decision-making protocol so that future denials assuming the experimental exclusion were irrefutable. I don't know what happened to the insured. Once the authorization was keyed into the information system, the claims submitted by the University of Nebraska Medical Center for this insured simply were paid.

About this time, the news was full of five cases being litigated on the west coast because of denials for autologous bone marrow transplant ABMT based on the insurance company's experimental exclusion. Two of them resulted in tens of millions of dollars in judgments. The uninformed, uneducated and the press labeled these outcomes as examples of managed care abuse and asserted that ABMT was not experimental because these companies had been successfully sued.

In reality, the three cases where the insurance company prevailed rested on the fact that a proper, consistent medical decision-making process was in place and had been followed. The requested experimental care was denied, and the appeals committee upheld the denial. The two successful litigations were not about the experimental status of ABMT. They were unfair claims practice lawsuits. There is no ERISA protection for unfair claims practices.

The central issue in these two cases rested on the fact that experimental care had been authorized for an executive's wife, but the same care denied for a low-paid employee. One judgment was for $80 million dollars. These insurance companies deserved to be punished and, in my opinion, got off easy.

On the East Coast, the same issues were boiling. In Maine, the state legislature mandated coverage of ABMT and high dose chemotherapy for the treatment of breast cancer. After millions of dollars were spent and untold lives shortened due to the procedure, long-term studies verified that the experimental treatment was no more effective than standard available care.

Benefit Denial and Back Pain: The Role of the Medical Director

A news story reporting an authorization request for a denied experimental treatment would grab headlines, but if the benefit denial could be made with absolute certainty, denial would be upheld. The number of these high profile determinations made by the medical directors was small compared to the number of UR authorizations handled by the nurses daily. Utilization review focused on hospital and facility admissions, length of stay, and on a limited number of high cost, frequently unnecessary imaging procedures.

For example, back surgery for a ruptured lumbar disk is a very costly procedure with an incidence that varies directly with the aggressiveness of the surgeons. Surgical outcomes are highly variable and more dependent on patient psychosocial factors than verifiable physical abnormalities. The medical literature reviews of imaging studies of the back verify that MRI and CT scans show half the population has bulging lumbar disks. A researcher would say lumbar imaging lacks both specificity and sensitivity as a diagnostic study.

Therefore, the imaging studies are not very helpful. In fact, they may be misleading regarding the medical necessity for back surgery. Much more than non-specific back pain was required to meet the standards. There were criteria for determining the medical necessity of doing an MRI or CT scan for several areas of the body commonly imaged.

The medical literature also confirms that most physicians do not manage back pain appropriately. Medical practitioners tend to overuse pain medications and "bed rest." Physical therapy is underutilized. Studies have shown that chiropractic care is more successful in limiting the length of disability and promptly returning people to work than our ubiquitous Allopathic Medicine.

EHIC required preauthorization of MRI and CT studies and the utilization review nurses had the standard criteria at their desks. I worked with the Provider Relations Department to develop a network of chiropractors and our HMO benefit package allowed several visits for chiropractic care without a referral authorization.

A relatively small number of high cost, frequently misused medical procedures and studies required preauthorization. Preauthorization was only feasible for those procedures and tests where solid, universally accepted criteria and standards of care, were available. Our UR nurses preauthorized procedures or studies based on criteria and standards of care developed by physician professional organizations (e.g., the AMA and physician specialty academies).

EHIC was not in the business of questioning everything the doctor ordered. High volume and low cost tests would be monitored by our information systems. By tracking the network provider's medical services by patient and by disease, cost of care comparisons for specific illnesses could be made. A rough estimate of the efficiency of our network providers could be made and reported retrospectively. Analysis of ongoing paid claims could also provide an estimate of outcomes by provider and by inference, the quality of care delivered. These data would later become the basis for the development of provider quality bonuses.

At this point, you should have a clear understanding of what an insurance company or HMO medical director is and is not. The medical director is a Doctor of Osteopathy (D.O.) or Medical Doctor (M.D.), usually with a board certification. The value the medical director brings to the HMO is training in, and understanding of, medical jargon and procedures, for the very limited number of high-cost services that the medical review department oversees.

The duty of the medical director is to have profound knowledge of the health care plan benefits, limitations and exclusions. General medical knowledge is important but communication skills are a necessity. The director must understand the insured's disease process and care proposed by the practicing physician. The community standards of care for the condition should be understood, but the critical skill needed is matching the physician's treatment plan with the generally accepted criteria and standards of care for the insured's medical condition.

The core task is to match the care plan with the medical standards and determine if the benefit plan supports authorization or denial of coverage.

The medical director is an interpreter or translator between the practice of medicine and the financing of proposed care by the contracted benefit plan. Medical director decisions *are not about what care should be provided—* they *are about justification of payment* for the care proposed or provided by the practicing physician. The medical director is neither an advisor to the practicing physician regarding diagnosis, nor medical consultant regarding the patient's plan of care. The medical director is not practicing medicine.

As medical director, I was also an administrator responsible for developing departmental policies and procedures. There is no comprehensive cookbook of managed care covering all possible benefit approval and denial decisions. The need for a common sense approach to medical practice was frequently communicated to partner network physicians. A common sense approach could help practicing physicians control costs, but common sense does not play well in a court of law when used for making insurance benefit determinations.

"Common sense" determinations simply reflect the application of the flawed global subjective memory-based decision-making process. This decision-making process was then (as it is now) the state-of-the-art of medicine for the majority of private physicians. This process is not very artful or complete. For defensible financial decisions, the established medical facts (as found in the patient's permanent record) must be matched to state-of-the-art universally accepted standards of care.

My experience and success with common sense medical decision-making was useless in my new career. I was no longer deciding what made good sense and was best for the diagnosis and treatment of my patient. I was now making financial decisions that had to comply with state regulations and the terms of the benefit contract. My communications, both written and verbal, were not just for the patient or attending physician. I would also be potentially communicating with the patient's attorney, a judge, and the little old lady in the second row of the jury box.

Medical Standards and Criteria

It was then that my quest began for the standards of care that would be critically important to the EHIC UR process. This was another spark of light toward the "greater epiphany" that was to come. This search for truth, justice and the American way was not easy. The Internet was not what it is today. Our legal department had a subscription to Lexus/Nexus, but the process of online research of applicable medical information was slow and tedious. We were using the original DOS operating system on very slow computers. The local hospital medical library was helpful in obtaining copies of available medical articles that focused on the standards of care. The practice of evidence-based medicine was known, but the scientific principles used in the discipline (for example, "Clinical Epidemiology") were not universally applied. There was much noise but little signal.

My search for available standards led to the US Preventive Services Task Force (USPSTF). From 1984 to 1989, this US Public Health Service program was charged with developing guidelines for medical services that were "preventive" in nature—in other words, services that could prevent future disease or provide screening mechanisms for early diagnosis when diseases are at more treatable stages. Before the publication of these standards, "screening" and "prevention" was whatever the doctor ordered. These published standards allowed fair, justifiable administration of the health care plan preventive service benefits.

The Task Force released the first report in 1989, the year the program was transferred to the Agency for Healthcare Research and Quality (AHRQ), under the US Department of Health and Human Services (HHS). As a result of this report and subsequent preventive service standard publications, the "banker's physical," including the yearly chest X-ray, began to fade away.

In addition to literature searches using Lexus/Nexus and the hospital library, I also attended certified medical education (CME) conferences. These are essentially trade shows held in large venues where medical researchers present clinical studies in lecture halls. The hallways and sometimes a grand ballroom are packed with rows of booths, rented by drug and medical device manufacturers. Insurance companies, HMOs and various medical service companies were also usually represented.

In 1989, Winifred Hayes delivered an hour presentation about her medical research company (Hayes, Inc.). She explained how medical standards are developed using clinical epidemiology and evidence-based medicine. Her organization also had a booth in the vendor hall. Wini was like a beacon of light over a sea of darkness. For a very reasonable fee (several hundred dollars per determination), Hayes, Inc. would research a procedure, treatment or drug and provide an effectiveness rating. The reports they produced would include the complete bibliography of the peer reviewed medical literature used to establish the "Hayes rating."

I had more experience with the stress of research and cost of developing defensible criteria than I care to remember. I understood the value of the Hayes, Inc. effectiveness rating service in facilitating appropriate benefit determinations for unusual, expensive services. This chance meeting was much more than a simple discovery of a service provider that offered accurate, defensible effectiveness opinions at reasonable cost. During our brief discussions, Wini clearly offered a profound understanding of the science of clinical epidemiology and evidence-based medicine, which was a key element in the success of her rating system.

The only physicians with the education, training and experience that qualify them to perform critical appraisal of the literature and develop standards for medical services are those trained in the science of clinical epidemiology. Physicians who are board certified in Public Health are in the small minority of qualified professionals. Wini had a staff of medical professionals and an advisory board of directors with special training in these disciplines.

I realized that most practicing physicians were clueless about evidence-based treatment standards or how clinical epidemiology could help them make better decisions about medical care for their individual patients. Some medical directors had a deeper understanding and awareness of these concepts but, like their comrades in clinical practice, were not well qualified to develop standards of care. My broad superficial awareness of these requirements helped me facilitate the development of a reasonable protocol for making benefit determinations regarding experimental procedures. I understood that I did not have the profound knowledge or the temperament to make medical criteria and standard development my life's work. My river of knowledge was wide but shallow and did not run very fast.

After returning to Green Bay, we signed a contract with Hayes, Inc. for access to the standards and criteria they had already developed. The contract also designated Hayes as our "special case" consultant to develop ratings for treatments or drugs on an *ad hoc* basis, and to assist in developing additional standards and criteria for those conditions. We continued to standardize our decision-making protocol and update all our existing managed care manuals. This would establish a justifiable, objective means of making decisions about coverage, but had the potential to improve outcomes for doctors who would follow the same standards and criteria for the treatment of their patients.

The First Epiphany—the Vision Develops

My quest for utilization review standards continued, resulting in my discovery of Dr. Lawrence L. Weed's work on the problem-oriented medical record. Until the late 1980s, I was unaware of Dr. Weed and his revolutionary philosophy, teachings and writings. Dr. Weed first published *Medical Records, Medical Education, and Patient Care: the Problem-Oriented Medical Record as a Basic Tool*[11] in 1969, the year of my internship at St. Luke's Hospital in

---

11 Weed, Lawrence L. (1969). *Medical Records, Medical Education, and Patient Care: The Problem-Oriented Record as a Basic Tool.* Cleveland: Press of Case Western Reserve University. (http://lccn.loc.gov/69017686)

Milwaukee. I had been trained before his teachings had any impact on the educational system that he decried.

He observed that our educational system of *memorization, regurgitation and certification* produced so-called expert decision makers, who, unfortunately, relied on the dysfunctional system of memory-based global subjective judgment when making their decisions. This fundamentally flawed decision-making process, combined with the paper storm of medical records, has resulted in the chaos and crisis we see today.

Looking back, the paper medical records in my Cudahy and Oklahoma Avenue offices and the paper charts I used at the hospitals certainly were not "problem oriented" using Dr. Weed's definition. Virtually all medical records then (as the majority are now) were paper documents kept in files at the individual doctor's office and at the insurance company. In other words, individual bits of medical information about the patient were filed, new results stacked atop old, and maintained according to its source (like lab reports, X-ray reports, consultations, surgical reports, etc.), in a paper-based, source-oriented record keeping system.

The architecture of the paper chart was the basis for the organization of data in the old, large insurance company legacy computer systems that store information in unrelated flat files. These computer files mimic the filing cabinets in back offices, even if they no longer take up the same amount of space. In other words, the source of the information determines its position in the paper medical record—and in computerized record systems today. For example, all laboratory reports are found in one section of the file while all X-ray reports are located in another. All consult reports may be in the back of the chart. Another section contains copies of hospital records (admission history and physical, discharge summary, etc.). None of these data are unified to create useful information about a patient's problem (e.g., "back pain").

The data in various source-oriented files are not inter-related to specific patient problems. The data are organized to maximize and increase the efficiency of billing for goods and services. Most of the information in the patient's chart documents the goods (e.g., medications, equipment, oxygen) and services (e.g., procedures, surgeries, doctors' visits) that have been delivered for a fee. Physicians practicing incident medicine document the diagnosis that justifies the treatment ordered or delivered during the office visit. The medical record makes the process of documenting services for collecting fees efficient. It is easier for the accountants to follow the money.

Paper charting evolved over time through the recommendations of specialty boards and requirements of state Professional Review Organizations (PROs). PROs instituted several changes (such as inclusion of a prominent list of allergies, current medications and diseases) to facilitate the "peer review" process. Peer review allows credentialed quality assurance professionals (a group of professional peers) to assess the physician's compliance with standards of care and billing.

However, the addition of these summary pages and standardizing source categories did little to improve the quality of care the physician actually delivered. Physicians were expected to know and apply the published medical care standards and criteria. Bits of medical information remained unrelated to each other and disconnected from the patient. The use of source-oriented paper charts impeded the delivery of patient-centered care and the development and implementation of problem orientation in patient records.

The development of inexpensive personal computers and relational database programs has facilitated the organization and presentation of the medical information any way the physician user wished to view it. The computer database programs allowed relating bits of medical information to each other and to the patient. However, most programs do not comprehensively coordinate or integrate the data, and most physicians, because they do not understand the potential power of electronic medical records, do not expect them to.

Dr. Weed was one of the first physicians to recognize both our medical record structural problems and the chaos caused by physician's applying global subjective memory (intuition) to medical decision making. He revolutionized the structure of medical records. He focused on the patient's problems connecting them to what the doctor ordered. He demanded the physician identify the goal of therapy, possible complications and expected outcome. He made *evidence-based medicine* operational in real time for the practice of medicine.

The Problem-Oriented Electronic Medical Record

A patient-centered or problem-oriented electronic medical record[12] (POEMR) focuses on the patient's problem by documenting the physician's critical thinking and decision making during the episode of care. The POEMR is structured to organize the physician's thoughts, document the physician's assumptions and provide the foundation for the application of medical decision support tools. The physician determines the patient's problem list through a detailed psychosocial history, medical history and physical exam. The physician develops a plan for each of the patient's medical problems that lists the following:

---

12 Weed, Lawrence L. (1991). *Knowledge Coupling: New Premises and New Tools for Medical Care and Education.* N.Y. Springer-Verlag. page 21

- Goal (expectations for the patient's health outcomes and resolution of problems)
- Basis for the problem statement
- Status of the problem
- Disability from the problem
- Symptoms and objective parameters to follow
- Treatments
- Further investigation to verify diagnosis or seek alternative options
- Possible complications

The office visit progress notes for each problem need to follow the SOAP format:

S: Symptomatic and subjective data (patient states, "I feel hot.")

O: Objective data (patient's temperature is 102°)

A: Assessment (fever of undetermined origin or FUO)

P: Plan for the next steps (blood and urine tests)

This charting system does far more than improve the quality of health care decisions negotiated between the patient and the doctor. It provides rapid accurate communication of the patient's unique medical problems, evaluation and treatments to any other medical professional with access to the chart. It clearly documents the basis for the physician's decision-making process.

I read all the relevant information I could find regarding his approach to medical education and practice. Dr. Weed identified a great truth, but seemed to be a dreamer in pursuit of the ideal. I understood his reality and believed in his dream, knowing that virtually all our medical delivery system problems would be solved in an ideal world that embraced his philosophy and implemented his tools.

Dr. Weed was the pioneer in the field of Problem-Oriented Electronic Medical Records (POEMR). The paper charting system he developed focused on the patient and the patient's problems. The introduction of relatively inexpensive personal computers (PCs) made it possible for him to develop an early electronic medical record, using the original DOS operating system. Following the original release of this early software, the development stalled. American physicians were not ready for problem oriented electronic medical records (POEMRs).

He also developed an informational database that could be related to and justify decisions made by the physician. In his words, he "coupled" patient problems with specific medical knowledge to facilitate appropriate decision-making. This was his approach to the problems created by "shoot from the hip" memory-based medical decisions. He is the founder of Problem Knowledge Couplers (PKC) Inc., a for-profit medical software company. They offer evidence-based medical knowledge software to support decisions physicians make in real time as they evaluate patient's problems.

I realized his research linking evidence-based medicine would help doctors diagnose and order treatment for their patients, and could dramatically cut physician error rates. This would have direct application to the EHIC utilization review process and would be a shortcut to help us develop our expanded system of medical standards and criteria. We do not live in an ideal world, but I knew his methods could at least help the EHIC utilization review process. I strongly believed that EHIC needed to contract with Problem Knowledge Couplers, Inc., Dr. Weed's development company, for a very cost effective "buy" rather than "build" decision.

I knew the science behind his work had very practical applications for the managed care industry. Therefore, I scheduled a pilgrimage to the metaphorical mountaintop in Burlington Vermont (Dr. Weed's home). There is a huge difference between believing in any particular philosophy and achieving profound understanding of its truth. Coming face to face with the visionary, looking into the "eyes of the prophet" as you listen to the "gospel," changes your view of the world.

My encounters with Larry Weed were not like seeing the light at the end of the tunnel. They were like emerging from the tunnel to a bright sunny day. It was a mind-altering experience. It was an epiphany. My past came together in the light of Dr. Weed's philosophy: my inclination to question authority and the "experts"; my experiences in and understanding of medicine; my knowledge of the perverse incentives of fee-for-service (FFS) reimbursement; and my training in quality improvement—all these experiences seemed to be leading toward a broader meaning in medical care. I gained a profound understanding of the shortcomings of our educational system in training medical professionals, and the inadequacy of the medical decision-making process. The path to reforming our broken health care system was through managed care procedures, standards, and criteria, continued quality assurance and empirical research. We cannot hope the ideal world will develop on its own or through expecting physicians and politicians to listen to their better angels.

My vision had taken shape—the future of health care would rely on linking empirical research results with creating standards in practice. This would not only provide better health care and outcomes for patients, but also would streamline and institutionalize efficiencies and cost-saving measures that would prevent the dangerous rise of the medical-industrial complex and its increasing stranglehold on the GDP. At this time, the shorter-term goals of this vision were:

- To contract with PKC, Inc. for development of medical decision support tools for the top one hundred human medical and psychiatric problems;
- To complete the development of the POEMR and integration with the PKC knowledge base;
- To develop and integrate a problem-oriented electronic medical record for the EHIC Medical Management Department to create records for all managed cases;
- To integrate the PKC medical knowledge decision support tools with the POEMR and the EHIC Badger claims processing system;
- To create a beta test site for the stand-alone system in the Green Bay Free Clinic by donating the hardware and installing the POEMR/PKC software system;
- To link the systems at the Green Bay Free Clinic beta test site with the systems used by the EHIC Medical Management Department—which would link into the Badger claims processing system;
- To provide the refined POEMR/PKC system with Badger links to EHIC partner physician clinics/groups; and
- To ultimately put the responsibility for proper utilization review in the hands of the EHIC partner physician clinics and groups.

Long term, this vision would more broadly link health care to these principles and make access to quality care the main goal of all people working in the system, from the orderlies and cafeteria staff to the medical professionals to the top execs and all the workers who helped process payments. In the short term, if EHIC could achieve these goals, our partner physician groups would have problem-oriented, electronic, computerized records linked to decision support tools. The use of these tools would reduce the number of full-time nurses staffing the utilization review function. What is the point of second-guessing the medical necessity of goods and services ordered by a partner physician who is practicing evidence-based medicine using universally accepted standards and criteria? The direct link to the home office Badger system would provide pre-approved electronic claims processing. As use of the remote systems grew EHIC could reduce the staff of the claims department. Ultimately, EHIC could evolve from an insurance company and HMO that used advanced computer systems to a software giant that sold a little insurance.

The revolution to build a better health care system would require a relentless push and series of small incremental steps until the goals were reached. I could start within my own realm of influence: EHIC. The problem-oriented electronic medical record (POEMR) and medical practice standards would have to be developed for the Health Maintenance Organization Utilization Review (UR), Case Management (CM) and Quality Assurance (QA) processes. Only then could criteria-supported decisions be linked to the Badger claims paying system.

Short term, I would need to convince the executives of EHIC that POEMR and standards for practice were necessary and should be linked through Badger—they would need to approve any financial backing to develop and make changes to the system. Once developed, the medical record and decision support tools would be migrated to the free clinic for beta testing and further development. The encounter data would be linked to the Badger claims adjudication system. Financial feedback and quality assurance reports could be returned to the free clinic board and volunteer physicians.

Once operational, the system would be offered to our partner physician groups. Use of the system would assure that efficient, appropriate and cost-effective medical decisions were made in real time at the point of service. This would eliminate the need for MCO utilization review and nurse reviewers. Uploading the record of billable patient care directly to the claims paying system would eliminate a significant number of claims processors. The system would be the application of technology with the human touch. Fee for Service reimbursement would be re-bundled into payment for episodes of care and disease state management (DSM) for populations of insured patients so the perverse piecework incentives would be eliminated.

I presented the business plan to our EHIC executive committee outlining incorporation of Dr. Weed's science into our Utilization Review (UR) and Large Case Management (CM) processes. I didn't discuss the vision's long-term potential, but stuck with the short-term, practical goals for EHIC. With this plan, EHIC would also provide Dr. Weed with a consulting contract for application of his software to the Free Clinic beta test site and the Badger managed care system. His contract would also reimburse quarterly presentations of his health care concepts and their application to the Badger medical management system at conferences. I secured approval to pay Dr. Weed one million dollars over three years to develop the standards of care with additional reimbursement for consulting fees.

I understood that Dr. Weed was a philosopher, academic and idealist, so the contract was written in the form of a grant. The contract specified Dr. Weed and PCK, Inc. would build a minimum number of "units" and gave EHIC non-exclusive access to the knowledge-based product. It called for him to present the EHIC criteria set and system applications at quarterly conferences and our yearly corporate meeting. It also specified that EHIC would pay Dr. Weed for the development of these criteria sets, but he would retain ownership of the knowledge generated. The contract was written to give Dr. Weed complete control over the process of knowledge generation, ownership of the knowledge, and control of its marketing to other companies.

Although Dr. Weed and I were in agreement about the end game, he was an idealist about the means; he could not rationalize getting into bed with a for-profit insurance company. I believe he trusted me personally, but felt the contract offer would have him make a deal with the dark side. Complete control and a virtually no-strings-attached million-dollar offer could not get Dr. Weed to sign the contract. The deal fell apart.

Despite this disappointment and the delay it would mean for the ultimate vision, I continued the slow development and refinement of medical management processes at EHIC. Dr. Weed continued to slowly recruit disciples to his philosophy as he and Problem Knowledge Couplers, Inc. (PKC) refined his undercapitalized system. My vision had taken form, but had to be put on the shelf, as other business needed attention.

Toward the end of the 1980s, the massive financial burden of developing the "Badger" computer program and a major recession resulted in a severe cash flow problem at EHIC. A reduction in force (RIF) was required to keep the company solvent. The company preserved the jobs of the front line workforce and reduced the numbers of middle management. Several Vice Presidents left the company to "spend more time with their families."

As part of the RIF, I was required to eliminate two out of the four managers in the Medical Management Department. From an emotional standpoint, this was one of the hardest tasks I would perform at EHIC. All the department managers were knowledgeable, dedicated hardworking professionals. My only consolation was the knowledge that as nurses they would have no problem finding work immediately.

Years later during one of President Obama's public relations visits to a major manufacturing plant, a worker mentioned she lost her job because of a "RIF." President Obama did not know what this was. When the worker said she had been laid off, he said, "Oh, like getting a pink slip." Not even the far right wing made anything of this conversation. As I watched I again lived through the emotions of the RIF meeting with my two managers at EHIC twenty years before. The incident also reminded me of the George H.W. Bush incident at a grocery store checkout counter. George the First had never seen laser bar code reader technology. The pundits raised the issue of being out of touch with the economy and the common person, but then I would not expect any president either to have been RIFed out of a job or to have purchased groceries in the prior twenty years.

Employers Health Insurance Company (EHIC) was purchased by Lincoln National Corporation (LNC) of Ft. Wayne, Indiana. LNC was a holding company that had several divisions. Lincoln National Life was the fifth largest insurance company in America. They had a financial service division and a reinsurance division. EHIC became part of LNC's Employee Benefits Division (EBD). EBD insured large employer groups and had purchased many smaller Administrative Services Organizations (ASOs) and HMOs across the country. John Cole, President of EBD, had been recruited from California and had brought the development of a massive relational database claims processing system with him. This meant Lincoln National Corporation EBD was going through the same managed care software development process as EHIC, but on a much grander scale.

Life went on for us in Green Bay. Norm and I continued to develop and manage the claims appeals process to assure conformance with state requirements and preservation of ERISA protection for the company. I helped manage the interface between the provider networks, Clinic Medical Directors and EHIC. I traveled across the state of Wisconsin with our provider relations managers performing regular site visits for financial efficiency and quality review.

Norm and I managed the development of a cost savings methodology for reporting productivity in utilization review and case management. This methodology was used to provide internal reporting to EHIC upper management. The same reports were summarized for external financial reporting to EBD upper management.

LNC/EBD also required weekly telephone conference calls for all medical directors for all company holdings—about 20 people including Norm and me. These meetings were held to coordinate and standardize the medical decision-making process and to develop additional medical standards and criteria for use by the various medical management operations across the country. We played the game but, given the difficulty of this task and the experience and training level of the group, I knew we were on mission impossible.

We had a great group of managed care medical directors. All were board certified in general medical specialties. Most were board certified in medical management and several had achieved their Master's degree in Business Administration. However, no one was trained in clinical epidemiology nor was anyone board certified in Public Health. These were insurmountable obstacles in making the vision a reality, even for our corner of the health care world.

Lincoln National Corporation/Employee Benefits Division: 1990 to 1991

Near the end of 1989, John Cole gave me an offer I could not refuse. He asked me to become the National Medical Director and Vice President of Medical Affairs for Lincoln National Insurance, Employee Benefits Division. Although we had limited contact with each other prior to my interviews and moving from Green Bay to Ft. Wayne, Indiana, I had developed a level of appreciation for and devotion to John that I had not experienced before or since. John was the only truly charismatic leader I have ever known. If John had said, "We shall storm the gates of hell" I would have asked, "When do we start?"

The Lincoln National Corporation (LNC) board of directors hired John Cole as the president and CEO of the Employee Benefits Division (EBD). The Board understood the need to transition EBD from the old reactive indemnity insurance model to the proactive managed care model. John had come to LNC/EBD with the massive database managed care information system he had started while working in California. The System for Managed Care (SMC) would eventually absorb EHIC's Badger database claims processing system.

My responsibilities as LNC/EBD Medical Director were similar to my duties at EHIC but at a much higher level. I had reported to Ed Elder, Vice President of Operations at EHIC. At LNC/EBD I reported to John Cole, the president of the division. Those who directly reported to me included the medical directors at EBD, who managed the local UR and CM functions and the corporate director of Quality Assurance. All other medical directors across the country were my "dotted line reports." In other words, their day-to-day activities were under the direction of their local business unit president or executive committee, but they looked to EBD, and my office, for direction and coordination of criteria development and implementation, and Quality Assurance activities. Their boss reported directly to my boss.

My job, on a national scope, was to develop and coordinate all medical knowledge, policies, procedures and workflows used by all LNC/EBD medical management departments. I was essentially a facilitator and managed a countrywide quality improvement process for all internal policies, procedures and benefit determinations for all LNC/EBD business units. This might sound like I had a big, important, powerful job, but in reality, the best job description for my position would be "Cat Herder." And I was at a level where the cats were not loveable, little kittens; they were hungry, and sometimes angry, lions and tigers.

Roadblocks to smooth operations as I transitioned into the position included the clash of corporate cultures, resentment of orders coming down from the home office, resistance to change and rejection of anything "not invented here." I learned a lot about big corporation and inter-corporation politics in a very short time. The medical directors soon realized that my intent was to help them get their jobs done, not micro manage their lives. As a Deming disciple, I believed my job as a director was to get the tools to the workers, then get the hell out of their way. Mutual respect was established and we could get on with our work.

Through phone contact and site visits, I discovered many medical management operations had out-of-date medical necessity and length of stay (LOS) criteria sets. Some criteria subscription renewals were as many as three years out of date, but the criteria vendors required yearly subscription renewal. In most cases, the medical directors knew this was a problem, but their direct bosses, as a cost cutting measure, had told them not to renew subscriptions to criteria publications. As a practical matter, LOS and most medical standards of care do not change in three years. Nevertheless, this did not excuse failure to honor their contract requirements.

Of greater concern was the lack of a defensible medical policy determination methodology across the entire country. Many of our medical directors developed policy for their business units the way most physicians practice incident medicine. They might shoot from the hip or ask the opinion of a board certified so-called expert. Policy and procedure manuals were not current or were completely absent. The medical directors understood the liability and public relations problem that using old criteria could present, and welcomed my efforts to update and standardize criteria sets.

I negotiated a contract with Hayes, Inc., to supply their effectiveness determination manual to our organizations and to develop special topic determinations for a negotiated fee. The medical directors reviewed and approved the Hayes manual at an early teleconference. The Hayes manual provided effectiveness ratings for a limited number of potentially high cost, complicated medical procedures. Hayes did not develop a complete, universal policy and procedure manual for EBD. The medical management department had the responsibility for this work. Our benefit policy development methodology for more common, less intense medical procedures relied on peer reviewed evidence-based medical information.

Our managed care business unit in Colorado employed a small group of medical professionals capable of supporting criteria development. I assembled a team of highly qualified professionals, including a trained medical librarian, to research criteria topics. The medical directors discussed and prioritized benefit coverage questions for development by this team. The Colorado research group gathered and assessed the relevant medical literature. I would develop a benefit policy proposal. The Colorado office distributed the information packets and proposed policy to all medical directors prior to our teleconferences.

Our medical directors reviewed the medical rational for and wording of the proposed policy determination. We developed final policy wording for recommendation to the executive boards of each local business unit. The local executive committee, with input from their compliance, legal and marketing personnel, would adopt or reject use of the policy. Because the development methodology was sound, no executive board ever rejected a policy recommendation. We developed over sixty benefit determination policies during my time at LNC/EBD.

The Japanese Visit Fort Wayne and Attention Paid to Quality Assurance

Shortly after we moved to Ft. Wayne, the executives attended a cultural sensitivity meeting. A Japanese company would be collaborating with LNC and we would be meeting some of their executives. We learned how to trade business cards and bow slowly from the hips while seriously studying your counterpart's card. The deeper the bow and the longer the contemplation, the more respect for the individual was communicated. After all my Deming training, I had great respect for the Japanese. His Total Quality Management (TQM)[13] methodology had turned their manufacturing segment into a powerhouse.

Although Deming did not promote "technological solutions," his work with Japanese car manufacturers, their workforce and their robot assembly systems led to the philosophy of "*Technology with the Human Touch.*" I believed Deming's emphasis on long-range planning meant this Japanese insurance company understood EBD's value as a major insurance provider with a sound business plan in the United States and were making an investment in the future. I did a lot of bowing and contemplating during the cross-cultural meetings.

Quality Assurance was getting a lot of press at this time. As part of HMO-enabling legislation, regulations were in place mandating assessment of quality assurance programs and documentation of outcomes. The National Committee for Quality Assurance (NCQA) had been established in 1990 with a grant from the Robert Wood Johnson Foundation. The organization held two-week training programs for interested, qualified physicians and nurses.

Both the government and NCQA focused on Quality "Assurance" rather than Quality "Improvement." There is no way to assure quality. Quality may be measured and improved but not guaranteed or assured. Initially, the focus of NCQA was on assessment and rating performance, not on process analysis

---

13 See Appendix.

and improvement. Pointing this out did not endear me to their instructors. For the most part, I went along to get along. It would take years for NCQA to evolve into a more Deming-like model, but eventually they also saw the light; by the late 1990s, both NCQA and the Centers for Medicare and Medicaid Services (CMS) would assess HMOs based on the effectiveness of their Quality Improvement programs.

In the meantime, it was my job to facilitate all our managed care operations in their transition from state insurance department review requirements to the NCQA model. This met with some resistance from the quality assurance nurses in a few backwater operations, but short discussions with their executives, legal and compliance departments and medical directors usually resolved any issues.

I directed the development of the criteria and methodology to evaluate transplant centers. Working with David Willis, our national Provider Relations Department, the committee I chaired credentialed over 125 programs, establishing our comprehensive transplant referral network. Key issues were survival time of the transplanted organ, survival time of the host (patient), and length of time the transplant team had been operational. The Provider Relations Department managed the cost-of-care through fee contract negotiations.

Another company had developed Centers of Excellence and trademarked the name. David Willis, the Assistant Vice President managing provider relations came up with the name "Centers of Distinction" (COD). In private, when we discussed life over a couple of beers, we affectionately referred to this project as "Cadavers on Demand." Medical people in general have a very dark sense of humor.

My home office team refined and implemented UR and CM cost savings reports to provide information that was more accurate to EBD senior executives. We streamlined and increased the effectiveness of the claims appeals process while preserving customer focus and the Employee Retirement and Income Security Act (ERISA) protections.

David and I also spearheaded the effort to establish a national formulary. I chaired the Pharmacy and Therapeutics Committee that developed the national HMO and PPO formularies and programs to incentivize physician compliance. David negotiated significant rebate dollars from the pharmaceutical manufacturers that produced the drugs listed in these formularies.

Years later, when Congress and George W. Bush enacted the Medicare Prescription Drug, Improvement, and Modernization Act of 2003 (MMA— effective on January 1, 2006), price negotiation with Big Pharma was excluded. I do not believe the prohibition was about preserving American capitalism, or the evils of socialized medicine, or drug companies not being able to afford future research. Just follow the money. Part D restrictions were all about power and money-driven politics.

Reform of our medical delivery system and my vision for how to accomplish it was never far from my mind. At EBD, I had the luxury of considering national implementation of such a program. I discussed my vision of the future and how we could make steps toward it using achievable goals with John Cole. In the long term, developing intelligent medical decision support tools would complement the System for Managed Care (SMC) massive relational database claims processing software under development very well. The ultimate administrative and medical cost savings would be huge. The income from licensing such a system would significantly and positively impact LNC shareholders.

Short-term, the project would be limited to medical criteria and an internal record system so it was doable without a significant change to our budget. I made a second attempt to partner with Dr. Weed. The contract parameters were similar, but his time the offer was five million dollars The partnership agreement specified that Dr. Weed would control the knowledge and, if EBD dropped the project, he would own the information and walk away with moneys paid. Once again, although we were trying to reach a similar end, Dr. Weed could not tolerate the means to this end. Despite my good relationship with him and my cajoling, it still meant collaborating with a for-profit insurance company. I secured approval from John Cole and the EBD Executive Committee to go ahead with our own development and build the system internally.

With significant cross-division cooperation and input from some very special and intelligent people, we wrote a formal business plan for developing an automated health care knowledge-based system to support medical decisions and clinical evaluations of provider practice patterns. During this process, on the recommendation of a close friend, I attended a two-week Certified Medical Education (CME) program for training in clinical epidemiology and critical appraisal of the literature. The program was held at McMaster University Michael G. DeGroote Medical School in Hamilton, Ontario. McMaster Medical School is one of the few institutions that stress clinical epidemiology, coordination of medical care and problem solving.

During my two weeks of intensive training (residing in an elder hostel student dorm), my river of knowledge got just a little wider and deeper. I knew that this training would help me be a much better manager of the people and process than a developer of the knowledge-based system. I did not know at the time that I was heading for the falls.

After I returned from McMaster University, the internal business proposal was presented to the EBD executive committee. With some modification,

Phase One was approved: we were authorized to begin recruitment of five teams to develop the knowledge base.

However, before we could get started, John Cole told me the project was on hold. Within several months, he told me LNC would sell all assets of the Employee Benefits Division, and I would be receiving outplacement services and a severance package. I felt like I was being carried toward Niagara Falls wearing only an undersized life jacket. He said it was very important I didn't share this information with the friends I had made working at EBD or friends and co-workers in other divisions of LNC. I couldn't tell the people I had recruited to work on the project who had become close friends. I was on the horns of the dilemma between loyalty to John Cole and close personal friendships. These friends could also be losing their jobs and would benefit from a head start finding work. I made the professional choice but lost several very good friends.

I walked out of the EBD building in the early fall of 1991 thinking, "It's not personal. It's only business." This was the first severance package of several to come. There was no multimillion dollar golden parachute for anyone. My severance package included psychological counseling (job loss being one of the major causes of depression), off-site office space for conducting my job search, and six months' salary and benefits extension.

I had no way of knowing the Japanese company, Dai-ichi Mutual Life, had purchased almost four and a half million shares of Lincoln National Corporation stock in 1990 and 1991. Dai-ichi was interested in LNC financial services and the stock purchase may have been more about raiding the corporation than establishing a long-term relationship. My belief that the Japanese had profound knowledge of continuous quality improvement was shattered.

The Japanese auto manufacturer Dr. Deming worked for in the 1950s has recently had significant quality issues. They lost their way concerning quality improvement. Perhaps too much good old American short-term profit orientation rubbed off when they started manufacturing cars in the USA.

Dai-ichi seemed to take the same short-term view. I believe they were interested in Lincoln National Reinsurance and Financial Services only. Most of the other divisions of LNC would eventually be sold off. It turned out to be a good business move for Dai-ichi and probably for the executives and big stockholders of LNC. The sale of the various divisions produced significant cash and, with the high-flying financial growth during the Clinton administration, the stock price of LNC Financial Services went through the roof. However, I was on the street, looking for a position with an organization willing to carry the vision forward.

CHAPTER 6:
The Wandering Medical Director

Fall in Ft. Wayne Indiana is a beautiful time of the year. Kathy and I lived on a hillside in a wooded area, several miles west of Interstate 69. The house was on eight acres, overlooking a small meadow, where a winding stream ran through a corner of our property. The weather had cooled; the leaves had begun to turn. We frequently saw small herds of deer crossing the stream into the woods beyond.

I left for work on a crisp Monday morning in early October, but this would not be like work days in the past. I would drive the same route, turning left off Hamilton Road onto Liberty Mills and, after a short stretch of Highway 24, onto Interstate 69. Driving north for several miles would bring the Employee Benefits Division Building of Lincoln National Corporation into view.

The windows where my office had been were visible, but my drive would no longer include exit 105, since I no longer worked at Lincoln. The daily drive would be a little farther down the road, but a lot longer in terms of emotional energy. An "off campus" office complex had been provided for the several managers and directors who had been terminated to "work." The out-placement consulting firm had rented this facility, with a secretary, mail service, copy machines, printers, phones and a facsimile machine.

If you closed your eyes and sat quietly, the place smelled and sounded like a real business. Real work was being done. All of us, with the exception of the secretary, were engaged in the full-time, all consuming occupation known as "the job search." Over half my severance package would be burned up before the next job offer came.

Several executive recruiters, with experience in the health care industry, were working on my placement. These people are essentially very highly paid matchmakers or "yentas." Due to their contacts with managed care organizations and insurance companies, they know when positions become available. They usually have a "stable" or portfolio of candidates suitable for a spectrum of positions in medical management.

Some large companies place executive recruiting firms on retainer. The recruiter "qualifies" or screens the potential executive. An applicant for an upper level management position does not get in the door for an interview without comprehensive vetting. These professionals also provide valuable services to the applicant. Resumes may be "tuned up" specifically for the targeted company. The applicant receives valuable information about the executives and the company prior to the interviews. Following the visit, the recruiter will contact the applicant for a "debriefing."

Between 1985 and the fall of 1991 I had experienced several flashes of enlightenment and a *major epiphany*. I understood that the central cause of the quality and cost crisis in the American medical care delivery system was the global, subjective, memory-based decision-making process. With a lot of assistance from some very bright people, a managed care plan to address the problem had been developed. Armed with profound knowledge of quality improvement and an absolute belief in the solution in hand, I was ready for the crusade. I needed to find a position with a large insurance company, with the financial resources to take on the cause and complete the reformation.

My choices for the first interviews were United Health Care in Minnesota and Anthem Blue Cross in Michigan. After discussions with the recruiters, my resumes were tweaked to emphasize the past accomplishments that would make me a better fit for the targeted companies. The recruiter told me I was in the final three candidates for the position with United.

My interviews with the medical management team at United Health Care went well. For interviews with the quality improvement team, I stressed my background training as an NCQA reviewer and in TQM. I held my own in intelligent conversations with the Information Technology Executives. As a believer in managed care, I was in accord with the medical directors in Utilization Review and Case Management. My last interview was with Bill McGuire, the COO of United Health Care. My assumption was that I would not have gotten this far if there were any strong objections to my candidacy.

The interview lasted about 20 minutes. Dr. McGuire seemed preoccupied and not well organized. We had little eye contact, and he spent most of the time staring out of his window as we talked about the goals he had for the company and his expectations regarding the open position. United Health Care selected one of the other candidates for the position. If the name "McGuire" sounds familiar, it should. Bill McGuire was paid $1.1 billion (yes, that billion, with a "B") when he left the company in 2006.

My interviews several weeks later at Anthem also went well but, once again, another candidate secured the position. After these two rejections, some soul searching was in order. Thinking about my interviews, it occurred to me I might have been too enthusiastic, especially when talking to the folks managing the technical and computer support systems. I had probably offered too much information and been too eager to push the envelope. I had forgotten the lesson of John the Baptist.

To secure a position I would have to be a "closet visionary." The free-fall after the bottom dropped out at LNC/EBD had ended. My resume was tuned for the interview with the administrator and medical staff at the Miami Florida Metropolitan Life office. The vision and most of my past life as a quality expert was pushed to the back wall of the closet behind the plain gray suits.

The MetLife home office in New York directed the functions of many regional offices. The MetLife Southwest Regional Office was in Atlanta, Georgia. One of the regional claims processing offices was in Tampa, Florida. The small MetLife managed care office in Miami performed only utilization review (UR) and some case management (CM). I projected the image of a medical director with concern for utilization management and a desire to faithfully follow the approved criteria manuals. They were looking for someone to "drive the desk" and I understood I would have to *go along to get along*. The job offer came and included a reasonable signing bonus, a moving package, and several months' living-expense allowance, but a cut in salary. I accepted the offer and, in January of 1992, moved into the Marriott Residence Inn at the west end of Miami International Airport, just north of the Dolphin Expressway.

Kathy stayed in Fort Wayne to prepare for the move and to keep the house in order for the real estate broker. The sale of our home would take some time since the housing market had made a steep downturn when EBD closed and the community lost many high paying jobs. Our fifty thousand dollar loss of equity would be offset some by the Metropolitan signing bonus. On the bright side, for thirty years, Kathy and I had been talking about moving to Florida, but career and circumstance had gotten in the way. Metropolitan had opened the door to a smaller room but a bigger life.

MetLife, Miami Florida: January 1992 to May 1993

I remember Saturday February 15, 1992, as if it happened yesterday. It was a warm, sunny day in Miami as I drove east toward South Beach on the MacArthur Causeway past the cruise ships moored in Government Cut. The Miami Boat Show had started, and I was on my way to the Convention Center to look at some *big boy toys*. My car windows were down and loud Cuban Jazz was playing on the radio. As I crested the top of the bridge connecting the McArthur causeway with the beach, a scene of incredible beauty unfolded before me, as the cacophony of horns from a thousand boats drowned out the music. I knew 1992 was the quincentennial year of celebration of the discovery of America, but did not realize how big the party would be in Miami.

Replicas of the Niña, Pinta and Santa Maria were sailing up Government Cut between South Beach and Fischer Island, flanked by Coast Guard and police rescue vessels. An armada of small boats, all blowing their horns, surrounded them. The Goodyear blimp was floating overhead and several slow moving biplanes, towing banners advertizing the Miami Boat Show, flew over the shore, beyond the low buildings of South Beach. Had I died and gone to heaven?

My transition from a high level medical executive position in one major corporation, to a job as a front line medical director for another major corporation, was stressful, but at the same time, liberating. It was a mixed bag: not altogether good or bad, just different. The move was from Fort Wayne, a small city of 250,000, to the "magic city" of Miami, the fifth largest urbanized area in the United States, where five million people lived. I had left the gray skies and frozen tundra of the north, for a sub-tropical paradise of sunshine and coconut palms.

I also left behind a high-pressure top management position, with responsibility for directing a large number of support staff. The Metropolitan position was on the bottom rung of the medical management ladder, with no direct reports. I functioned like an independent contractor, but with salary and benefits. The quiet, fifteen-minute commute, with three stop signs, through a rolling wooded Indiana countryside, was replaced by a forty-five minute crawl, in stop-and-go bumper-to-bumper traffic, surrounded by cars driven by crazy people. Nevertheless, the traffic did not bother me. Overall, I had made a good decision.

Almost overnight, my high school level typing skills saw a vast improvement. My speed went from twenty words per minute, to greater than fifty. The process of sitting at a computer terminal, wearing a telephone headset while talking to physicians, and typing their comments and my rational for decisions into the computer, improves typing speed quickly. Our office used dumb terminals connected online with the mainframe claims processing system in Tampa, Florida. Our medical authorization or denial decisions would determine how the Tampa office adjudicated managed care claims.

As Senior Medical Director for South Florida Operations, I reported to Dr. Duvie, the Florida Managed Care Operations Director. Dr. Duvie had been brought in from New York City to build new business. He worked with the sales and marketing departments toward this purpose, and with the provider relations team, he worked to facilitate contracting with new providers. His focus was mainly outside the office. A second Medical Director, Dr. Kay Serah, also reported to Dr. Duvie. The Director of the UR and CM, Nurse Hatchet, reported to Dr. Duvie, and was the Office Manager.

Working Across Corporate Stovepipes Can Endanger Your Career

Quality Assurance and NCQA review were the educational topics of several monthly office staff meetings. My presentations covered the Florida regulatory requirements, but also stressed a "Deming" quality improvement management style, that mainly seemed to be received with, at best, indifference—people were not ready to listen to or embrace quality improvement innovations. On several occasions, during the spring and summer, I assisted with the home office effort to prepare for the National Committee for Quality Assurance certification review. The state reviewers scheduled the on-site visit to our Miami office for the fall of 1992.

It turned out the Medical Director for Quality Assurance at the Metropolitan Life home office in Manhattan was Dr. Paul Bluestein, a friend from a past life. I met Paul during NCQA training and we attended some of the same managed care educational conferences. My NCQA training made me a valuable resource to the company, serving as an internal consultant to the Regional Quality Managers Committee (located in Tampa). I served as the *lead reviewer* for internal NCQA preparatory site visits. These prep visits were like mock disaster drills. The team managed to assure every site was prepared. All Metropolitan managed care sites complied with the state mandated quality review requirements.

Unfortunately, no good deed goes unpunished. The Director of the South Florida Medical Management Office did not appreciate my cross stovepipe quality improvement activities. Perhaps Dr. Duvie felt threatened by my contact with Paul in New York. Alternatively, given his management style, these cross-functional support activities may have simply made him uncomfortable. Our office manager, Nurse Hatchet, being an old school head nurse, also did not appear comfortable with conversations about Deming's recommendations regarding management support for the people doing the work. The two of them would prove to be formidable foes.

It had become apparent that both Dr. Duvie and Nurse Hatchet were comfortable in their organizational stovepipe, and were top down micro-managers. This management style, sometimes referred to as "Taylorism," is easy to identify for anyone with minimum training or experience in Quality Management. This style had not been pushed to the extreme of workplace dehumanization for the rest of the MetLife team, but management was not much interested in input from the worker bees.

It is a common management style in very large corporations and all levels of government with multiple separate *stovepipes* of functionality. Stovepipes are separate defined functions within organizations having allocated budgets and chains of command composed of executives and managers. For example, the executives and managers in each of the different areas of design, engineering, production, claims processing, finance and sales stovepipes may severely restrict communication up and down the chain of command and may completely block cross-functional communication. Fortunately, most failures of cross-functional communication result in only waste of money. Sometimes the failure of cross-functional communication may be disastrous. Several years ago two United States Marine helicopters were shot down over the Kurdistan "No Fly Zone" by American Air Force Jet patrol planes. Air traffic control for the separate branches of the service had not communicated properly resulting in this tragic loss of life to friendly fire.

Many large progressive corporations have addressed this communication problem. Most have centralized functions that break down the barriers between stovepipes. Examples of centralized functions that facilitate communication are human resources, regulatory compliance, legal and quality improvement. The degree of support provided to these functions by upper management and the board of directors determines the effectiveness of these centralized functions and, ultimately, the effectiveness of the organization.

In any event, Dr. Duvie let me know he did not want me doing anything other than driving the UR desk in South Florida. He suggested my employment position was tenuous. In an instant, my respect for, and trust in the man was gone. My only option was to keep my head down and do exactly as he had instructed. I fully understood that doing *exactly* as a micromanaging boss instructs absolutely assures failure. However, there was no other option. Proverbs such as, "Once bitten, twice shy," and, "Fool me once, shame on you; fool me twice, shame on me!" are rules to live by in the corporate world, where trust is everything. My ass had been bitten once. It was not going to happen again.

Our conversation clarifying my duties did not qualify as a "performance review," or "step one," in a disciplinary process, as defined by corporate policies and procedures, but I understood the threat such a conversation with a boss imposed. Dr. Duvie did not understand the significance of our *clarification conversation*, but I certainly did, and treated it as initiation of the disciplinary process. I contacted the MetLife Corporate Human Resources by email, and requested a copy of the multi-step disciplinary policy.

The fact that our discussion of duties did not comply with corporate policies, and could be interpreted as a violation of them, did not make me feel better. For the next several weeks, every conversation with Dr. Duvie regarding my duties was documented. Several of his directives and clarifications of my duties seemed to be in direct violation of state and federal workplace regulations and MetLife policies. I acknowledged every verbal directive in an email within minutes or hours. I responded to his specific directions regarding work performance improvement by individual emails, with assurance of my cooperation and absolute compliance. I provided a blind copy of all these email communications to my contact in the Human Resource Department.

Copies of all emails were printed and taken home for my files. Because he gave limited feedback regarding written communications, I knew he rarely reviewed his own email. He was fond of saying, "You can't make an omelet without breaking some eggs," and must have been off breaking eggs instead of looking at his inbox. On the rare occasion when he provided written directives, I responded immediately by email with a plan for my compliance. After about six weeks of my being a "model corporate citizen," the Atlanta regional office director summoned Dr. Duvie for a management conference.

Within days of his return, he called me into his office, where he congratulated me on the fine work I had been doing and gave me an excellent performance evaluation. We never discussed any disciplinary issues and, in effect, declared an unspoken truce. Had he been called to Atlanta for a "Come to Jesus Meeting"? Possibly, but in any event, our superficial professional relationship changed for the better. However, trust would never be restored.

Hurricane Andrew: August 1992

On Sunday, August 24, 1992, shortly after this metaphorical trip to the woodshed, Hurricane Andrew hit South Florida. The devastation was widespread and electrical power was out in Miami for several weeks. It was a wakeup call. Kathy and I did not know much about tropical storms. We were living in a rented fourplex in King's Creek, just north and west of where the Palmetto Expressway crosses over Kendal Drive. Kathy had driven down with our son who would begin his Master's work in Business Administration at the University of Miami that fall semester. We braced the mattresses against the windows and slept on the floor, under the stairway, behind the couch. Mark slept on the couch. The building creaked and shuddered, as the roots of surrounding large trees were broken when the howling wind ripped them from the ground. Fortunately, the storm did not breach the building and no one from our complex or the MetLife office was injured or lost.

Prior to Hurricane Andrew, Kathy and I had spent a few days looking for the Florida dream home on or near the water. I drove our real estate agent crazy looking for a moderately priced home, located within 45 minutes to an hour from the MetLife office. Prices of homes on the water in Miami were financially out of reach, but properties in Key Largo could fit our needs and budget. After a long day at the office, a pleasant drive home in the evening, down the *18 Mile Stretch*, and over the Jewfish Creek Bridge at the Intra -Costal Waterway (ICW), would be just what the doctor needed, or that's what I thought before the hurricane.

Hurricane Andrew changed our view of this tropical paradise. We decided direct access to the ocean was a lot less important than direct access to a four-lane evacuation route. That fall we purchased an updated 1950s classic Florida pitched-roof home, just to the east of US 1, near the southern terminus of the Palmetto Expressway. The place had survived Andrew with minimal damage. MetLife was a forty-five-minute drive with the sun at my back both morning and evening. It would be our home for the next ten years.

Shortly after the hurricane, I made contact with Dr. Duvie and suggested that the medical directors and several nurses could set up a temporary UR and CM operation in the Tampa Claims Office. This would allow continuing medical management UR activities, but Dr. Duvie chose to shut down operations until the power was restored. This would take several weeks. All employees were, in effect, on a paid vacation. Other MetLife UR offices would manage our load.

By the beginning of September, the office was up and running once again. I was back driving my desk, feeling a little beaten up, but having a deeper understanding of the dynamics of our little South Florida office. The rest of the office suffered as well. Workplace moral was never better than mediocre, but now it was at an all-time low. What had been a moderate degree of employee turnover in the professional staff would soon grow significantly. Within a year, this would work to my advantage.

Managed Care and Administrative Issues: Lessons in Cost Containment

One of the responsibilities of my position was to assist the sales division in presenting managed care concepts to large national accounts (e.g., Mobile Oil, National Can, etc.). At various times, I was directly responsible for medically managing several major local accounts (e.g., Harris Corporation, Dade County School Board). I remember listening to the Dade County School

Board (DCSB) meetings broadcast on one of the Miami Public Radio stations on a Wednesday evening. Although the discussions could have provided teachers and staff an important "heads up" regarding health coverage issues with MetLife, the radio broadcast was definitely a cure for insomnia. Most educators lean left toward the more progressive end of the political spectrum, and the DCSB Metropolitan Health Care Plan reflected this, providing the insureds with a generous benefits package. We met with the DCSB Human Resource representatives once a month to discuss any problems they identified with general benefit and coverage issues. The Metropolitan Provider Network was mature and well established in Miami, so there were usually no administrative problems to discuss.

MetLife's relationship with Harris Corporation was an entirely different matter. The company is located in Melbourne, Florida, at the southern end of the "space coast," and is the largest employer in town. Harris is a high tech communications company, employing about fifteen thousand people, supporting the great majority of workers and their families in the area. It is an important Defense Department and NASA contractor. The workforce consisted of highly educated and trained, very intelligent folks. As you can imagine, because of their industry and clients, most of the employees leaned to the right politically, toward the more conservative end of the political spectrum.

In order to keep the costs of business competitive, Harris needed to get a handle on health care expenses. To do so, the company was transitioning from an indemnity, fee-for-service (FFS) health care plan to a managed care plan. Harris requested that MetLife build a network of providers for this product. Building a network of providers for this 900-pound gorilla was not a difficult task for the most part. Between the goodwill they garnered in the community and the contacts they had with important players, many inroads were available for MetLife to work more effectively. Harris provided an extraordinary amount of community service and support. Some executives served on the board of directors of the hospital, and many were the friends of the physicians and clinic administrators in town. The hospitals and clinics came on board and acquiesced to the fee schedule, utilization review program and balance billing restrictions.

Virtually all the providers in Melbourne cooperated with the program. The radiologists were the only exception. It seems there was only one radiology group in town, and they were a cartel. Executives at Harris pressured the administrators at the hospital where the radiology group had offices. This tactic had no effect. To be fair, hospital administrators are not good at pressuring staff physicians for any purpose. Such pressure rarely works to the benefit of the hospital. The hospital administrators have essentially no leverage.

When it was clear to Harris that the radiology group would not be cooperative, the company provided their employees with a solution. Harris initiated a demonstration "skunk works" project that involved electronic transmission of imaging studies performed at one location to another location for reading. I may be making this up, but I seem to remember the transmissions were from Melbourne, Florida, to California. This may be an example of one of the earliest long distance transmissions of such data. It didn't take the Melbourne radiologists long to understand the wisdom of cooperating rather than getting into a pissing contest with an international high tech communications company.

None of MetLife's large employer groups ever interfered with utilization review or individual benefit decisions made by the medical management department. Large employers have human resource, legal and compliance departments that understand the consequences of violating patient privacy laws and losing ERISA protections. Our medical management efforts resulted in lowering the number of inpatient hospital utilization by 100 days per 1000 lives covered. Significant reductions in the cost of outpatient services were also accomplished. The providers were catching on. Our efforts to correlate clinical epidemiology and objective, peer-reviewed medical criteria with benefit authorization requests seemed to be improving efficiency and quality. Payment authorization denials for medically unnecessary services had moved the local providers to a more conservative style of managing their practice.

During the fall, Dr. Duvie seemed to be having problems functioning within the bounds commonly set by large corporations. The MetLife Atlanta Regional Office asked Dr. Duvie to stir things up in South Florida; making omelets by breaking eggs was his specialty, after all. As the year progressed, omelets were nowhere to be seen, and Dr. Duvie started to act more as if he was walking on eggshells. He was not much of a corporate animal. I was very much a corporate animal, and watched his growing frustration with interest.

The 1992 election campaigns were engrossing. I felt George H.W. Bush had done a good job as President, even though the economy was having some difficulty. I liked what Ross Perot had to say, but realized most of the country would not think he was making sense. I voted for President Bush, but understood Clinton would probably win, because Perot would have siphoned off Republican votes. In any case, it did not seem to matter which party controlled the White House since the Republicans in Congress would maintain the status quo.

As the holidays approached, the Miami MetLife Managed Care Office plodded along, carrying on the day-to-day activities of utilization review and some case management. The monotony of the standardized authorization process continued, broken only by the occasional remarkable case. The UR nurses continued to authorize benefits for services that met the standardized criteria and the terms and limitations of the contract. Dr. Serah or I received those authorization requests failing to meet the standards for discussion with the practicing physician.

A nurse delivered a small stack of medical director referrals to my office on an hourly basis. These referral slips would document the MetLife case number, provider name and phone number. I would key in the case number, review the UR nurse comments and call the provider to discuss the payment authorization request. Many times special mitigating circumstances or complexities were found, allowing us to approve the benefit authorization. Sometimes the physician's documentation of the patient's findings failed to meet the medical criteria and standards that would justify benefit authorization, and benefits would be declined. Most decisions were clear and easy to justify based on reasonable standards and allowable exceptions.

Witnessed Phone Conversations and Flaming Gapers

For the gray areas where standard criteria did not seem to apply or the facts did not absolutely fail to meet the criteria, I would nearly always approve the benefit after a short conversation with the insured's physician. Occasionally a physician (or office nurse) would go on a rant abusing one of our reviewers. The UR nurses would deliver the medical director authorization request to me, and describe the conversation with the provider's office personnel. I would ask the reviewer to stay in my office to witness the return call (using my speakerphone) if even a minor cross interaction might occur during my call. A little paranoia went a long way under these "cover your assets" (CYA) circumstances.

If a very stressful situation were anticipated, I would consider a "two-witness call back," and ask a second nurse to witness the call. I would enter my log of the conversation with the provider into the comment section of the mainframe case file. Quotation marks set off the provider's comments. I would note the nurse witnesses and document the authorization basis for the decision (criteria met or not met). The reviewer(s) proofread my computer entry for accuracy of content. Once the "enter" key was pressed, the comments became part of the permanent electronic record and could not be changed. We could add comments to the file on new pages, but the original information could not be altered.

Several examples of witnessed callbacks come to mind. A neurosurgeon's office had called requesting an MRI of the back for an insured patient. The office nurse did not provide any information that would justify the medical necessity for the procedure, so our review nurse informed the office nurse approval of the procedure required a doctor-to-doctor conversation. Apparently, the physician heard half the conversation, picked up the phone, and went on a rant about the evils of managed care and generally abused our review nurse.

Sean Kean, my favorite orthopedic surgeon and a colorful Irish immigrant from my early career, classified doctors who exhibited such behavior "flaming, gaping, assholes." We shortened the phrase for use in polite company to "flaming gapers." I usually reserved such a designation until gaining enough experience with the individual to justify the title. From the description of the conversation, it seemed a one-witness conversation was in order.

The assumption was made that the doctor was simply having a bad day. When I called back, with the nurse reviewer in my office, the provider was calmer, but still on a minor rant. He demanded to know my qualifications. When told I was board certified in Family Practice and Medical Management, he demanded to speak to a board certified neurosurgeon. Our conversation from this point went something like this:

Me: "Surely, your mother is very proud of having a board certified neurosurgeon for a son, but this is not about you, and your board certification, or me, and my board certification. It is about your patient's problem." This comment shocked the doc into a few milliseconds of silence, which allowed me to explain the situation to him.

Me: "Please look at your patient's chart for your list of findings. The medical necessity for the MRI was not established, based on information we have been given regarding your patient, using the medical necessity criteria developed by your specialty organization. Perhaps our reviewer, or your nurse, missed something in your patient's chart?"

After a few seconds, the good doctor said gruffly, "Well, I have noted A, B & C, but it looks like X & Y have not been documented."

Me: "It sounds like you have the criteria nailed. MetLife uses the same criteria established by your specialty organization and from the orthopedic surgeons, to determine medical necessity for the MRI. Does your patient also have X & Y?"

Him: "Yes, my patient has A, B, C, X & Y. I have been having a very busy day and didn't chart the information."

Me: "OK, I'll approve the requested payment authorization. I'm sorry for the inconvenience and hope your day improves."

The neurosurgeon was not a "flaming gaper." He was just an overworked specialist who had gotten a little behind in his charting, and bent out of shape because he believed managed care administration would hassle him unduly—a perception he likely formed based on TV ads and griping with other docs over beers, not personal experience. There would have been no problem if the information had been in the patient's chart. Had the neurosurgeon properly charted this encounter at the time he saw the patient, the benefit authorization would have taken our respective nurses a minute or so. Because he did not complete the patient documentation, his day was more stressful.

In addition, without our conversation, his paper charting would have remained incomplete. Of course, this would only be important to the physician if this patient had a bad outcome and a malpractice lawyer started asking questions regarding justification for the procedure. A Medicare or Medicaid review of a sample of this provider's charts could reveal insufficient documentation of medical necessity for care delivered, prompting the regulators to demand repayment or trigger a full fraud investigation of his practice. In reality, proper charting is about quality patient care. Reimbursement and malpractice mitigation are distant second and third priorities.

The conversation did illustrate the misconception most physicians have regarding managed care. The interaction between the practicing primary care or specialty physician and the health plan medical director is not about professional training, certifications, qualifications, or the size of either doctor's memory banks. As the MetLife Medical Director, I was there neither to second-guess his judgment nor to offer a consultation about the medical condition of his patient. My job was not to offer alternative tests or treatment plans. I was there to establish if medical standards and criteria were or were not met, and to authorize or deny benefit payment.

He did not need an equally educated and trained super specialist to discuss the value of an MRI for his patient. He knew the standards for benefit authorization. His patient actually met the standards. He had simply failed to document all the evidence justifying the procedure in his patient's chart.

The medical directors often denied authorization for payment for MRIs. There would always be excuses for why the study or procedure was "needed." Many times, it simply boiled down to what the patient or doc demanded and wanted, regardless of the signs, symptoms and findings that would justify medical necessity and benefit payment. Such payment denial determinations are not examples of an insurance company, an administrator, a nurse, some bureaucrat, or the government getting between the patient and the doctor, as many people assume. Managed care payment denials represent the application of clinical epidemiology and evidence-based medical standards to evaluate payment requests for medical services.

Only a relatively small number of frequently misused, high cost procedures are subjected to this scrutiny. When the criteria and standards are met, authorization is approved, within the terms and limitations of the benefit plan. When not met, authorization of the benefit is denied. The physician and the patient determine if a test or procedure is *done*. The Utilization Department determines if the test or procedure is a *covered benefit* that the insurance company will reimburse.

Another Necessary Allegory: Uncle Sam and Your New Shoes

Although seemingly straightforward, these concepts have been twisted by some and ignored by others. An allegory may be helpful to understand the concept. Imagine that you have sore feet. Your old shoes were comfortable, but now seem to be causing you pain. You think you might need a new pair of shoes. If new shoes are necessary, your Uncle Sam has offered to pay for them at the Discount Shoe Outlet. If you need socks, he will pay for up to six pair per year, regardless of whether you want new shoes or not. However, he wants to be called if you plan to purchase a pair of shoes to decide if he will pay for them.

Uncle Sam knows you wear a size 10, doublewide. After driving to the Discount Shoe Store in the mall and talking with Mr. Scrolls, the Discount Shoe Outlet Manager, about your sore feet, he examines your shoes. The manager determines your shoes need polishing and that your insoles are hard, and need to be replaced. Mr. Scrolls recommends that only Chillin' insoles are needed, not brand new shoes. The Chillin' insoles and pack of six pair of white crew socks are added to your basket. Uncle Sam will pay for these without a phone call.

But wait! Walking into the store you saw a display of Italian loafers. After you ask about the shoe display, the manager consults a commissioned salesperson regarding your desire for Italian loafers. The sales consultant fits you with a pair of Italian loafers that are a little "snug," being too short and too narrow, but they are the only pair close to your size. Although these shoes do not fit and could cause you additional pain, you *want* them so you will *look good*.

You are also looking forward to showing off your fancy new shoes and endlessly talking to all your friends about the fitting process. Your salesperson will pocket a substantial commission, hence he is motivated to sell you the full price Italian loafers. He quotes Billy Crystal playing Fernando on Saturday Night Live saying, "It is more important to look good than to feel good!"[14]

However, when the manager calls your Uncle Sam to authorize the purchase, he has to admit only new insoles are needed. Uncle Sam will pay

---

14 See http://www.nbc.com/saturday-night-live/recaps/#cat=10&mea=396 &ima=92203 for a clip of this character.

for the Chillin' inserts and six pair of socks. If you decide to purchase the shoes, the cost will be entirely out of your pocket. You make the prudent decision and leave the store with Chillin' insoles, new socks and happy feet. Discount Warehouse Shoes bills your Uncle Sam directly. The pain in your feet goes away.

The Two-Witness Conversation and the Ninth Commandment

Not all benefit authorization challenges can be solved quite so easily. One "two-witness case" came from a female chiropractor who requested benefit authorization for manipulation a two-year-old toddler with a stiff neck. When the UR nurse delivered the referral slip, I had a flashback way back to the two-year-old child with almost imperceptible stiffness in the neck that turned out to be meningitis. Immediate referral to Milwaukee Children's Hospital had saved that child's life. I could not imagine that any chiropractor would consider manipulating the stiff neck of a child this young.

I called an additional nurse into my office as a second witness and called the provider back immediately. The information about the toddler was alarming. Several hours before seeing their chiropractor, the parents had noticed the child had neck stiffness and irritability. A chill ran down my spine. I told the provider (Dr. Wackumcrackum) she should consider recommending that the parents take their child to their pediatrician or the emergency room. The consequences of delay in diagnosis and treatment could be devastating for the toddler and the family.

I additionally mentioned the malpractice liability for the chiropractor could be significant if the child had early meningitis and the diagnosis was missed ("failure to diagnose" is a substantial liability for any provider). However, the fine line between raising the possibility of terrible consequences for the toddler, family and provider, and recommending a plan of evaluation, or treatment, could not be crossed. I did not require this action. I was not practicing medicine. I was administering a benefit contract and making reimbursement decisions.

The provider was informed that a blanket referral would be logged into the computer system to authorize any referral to any provider, in or out of network. I would ensure that no administrative processing would delay medical evaluation and care for the child. I believed this scenario might be a life-threatening emergency for the child, and would not let any insurance issues hold up proper care. Nevertheless, I could do no more. The authorization logged into the mainframe approved payment for any care within 72 hours. Such a blanket authorization would also approve benefit payment for any chiropractic care, should Dr. Wrackumcrakem ignore the danger. I do not know what ultimately happened to the child; I was only able to provide for any care the physician deemed necessary and hope they chose to do the right thing.

The patient medical information, statements by the chiropractor and me, and the names of the nurses present were logged into the file. As a benefit administrator, I could only hope that the provider had managed the toddler's medical care efficiently and effectively. Our team went back to our administrative functions, and it was back to business as usual. Several weeks later Dr. Duvie called me to his office regarding a "very serious matter." Nurse Hatchet seemed to have a smirk on her face when I walked past her desk on the way to see him.

Dr. Duvie produced a member service complaint log printout. It was from the parent of a two-year-old child, regarding statements made by the MetLife Medical Director (me). He slid his cheater reading glasses down to the end of nose, as he began, "The member states they were informed by their chiropractor, Dr. Wrackumcrakem, that the Miami Medical Director…" Dr. Duvie was not good at masking his enjoyment when trying to play the "gotcha" game. Remembering the case, I was more than happy to play along. He continued, "…Dr. Strube said, 'I hope the child develops meningitis and you get sued for malpractice!' Well…what do you have to say for yourself?"

I took a long pause to ponder what Dr. Duvie had said, while trying to hold a sincere look of puzzlement on my face. Dr. Duvie inquired, "Well?" Finally, looking as if a light had come on I replied, "I think I remember the case, and I am mortified that Dr. Wrackumcrakem could have so badly misinterpreted what transpired." The 1965 rock recording of "Please don't let me be misunderstood" by the Animals[15] began playing in my head. I asked him to pull the file up on his computer, so he could view the comments. He needed a little help accomplishing this.

The sections logging the conversation and documenting the names of the nurses witnessing the interaction were listed. I said with a grin, "That's my story, and I'm sticking to it. Do you want me to ask the nurses to come to your office now?" Dr. Duvie, with what sounded to me like a tone of disappointment in his voice, responded, "Thank you, I'll take it from here." The nurses were interviewed. The accuracy of the conversation, as documented in the computer files, was confirmed. The issue was never brought up again.

---

15 The Animals. (1965, US). "Don't Let Me Be Misunderstood." MGM Records. Writers: Bennie Benjamin, Gloria Caldwell, & Sol Marcus. Producer: Mickie Most. Retrieved on December 26, 2010 from http://en.wikipedia.org/wiki/Don%27t_Let_Me_Be_Misunderstood.

My preference is to believe that Dr. Wrackumcrakem misinterpreted our conversation and simply used poor judgment when discussing our interaction with the parents. The assumption should always be that people, in their business and personal lives, are operating in good faith. However, discovering someone has attempted to burn you, or play you for the fool, changes the relationship forever. MetLife Member Services Department would clarify the misunderstanding with the insured patient, and would copy Dr. Wrackumcrakem with the communication. The next conversation between the parents and chiropractor must have been very interesting.

There have been times when practicing physicians have altered patient charts and maliciously misrepresented conversations with utilization review nurses or medical directors, but this probably was not one of them. Most physicians and patients do live by the Eighth (Catholic/Lutheran) or Ninth (Anglican/Other Christian) Commandment, "Thou shall not bear false witness against thy neighbor."

MetLife Reorganization and Discovering the Geek Shall Inherit the Earth

Not long after the office Christmas party at the end of 1992, Dr. Duvie announced he would be leaving MetLife and moving back to New York City. Nurse Hatchet may have been the only member of the office staff that considered his departure regrettable.

MetLife was undergoing some organizational and product changes at this time. I was called to Atlanta for a conference with the MetLife Regional Director of Marketing, Frank Lee Skarlott. Although I was hoping this was an opportunity for advancement because the "marketing stovepipe" was the most important business unit in the company, I was wary of a potential downside to the meeting because of the reorganization that was underway.

I hastily put together a short business plan for the reorganization of the Miami office, carefully addressing the morale issues, and I got on the plane for Atlanta. The meeting was short and not very sweet. I met with Frank and his Director of Florida Marketing Operations, Hugo Orygo.

It became immediately apparent that Nurse Hatchet was very well connected with the Atlanta Office and I was on the wrong end of a *two witness* meeting. These two marketing people were not interested in the reorganization or morale of the Miami Office. They wanted to know if I could *get along* and *work with* Nurse Hatchet. It was obvious that if they were forced to make a choice between us, Nurse Hatchet would stay. There was no way I would give her the satisfaction and give them an excuse to make this choice.

When asked about my professional relationship with the Office Nurse

Manager, I replied, "We do have some minor differences in management style, but it is my belief that she is a very professional and competent manager. No matter how the Miami Office is reorganized, we will work well together." They were not impressed with my proposed Miami office organization chart keeping her in command of the nurses. They seemed skeptical, but I had not empowered them to do me any harm.

During my return to Miami, there was ample time to think about this encounter. Why would a nurse manager, in a small satellite medical management office, be this important to the Regional Director of Marketing? I doubted she had any pictures of these guys with sheep. Although I believe it is more of a problem with medium-to-large privately held companies, or small corporations, not national corporations like MetLife, it occurred to me that, in the past, people in the marketing stovepipe may have attempted to "influence" benefit determinations. It was not uncommon for people at the top of the insurance company heap to contact their health insurance marketing rep to reverse an authorization denial for themselves or members of their families. The local rep would get to the regional manager, who would pressure the Vice President of Marketing, who would lean on the claims or managed care department, to authorize payment. This happened to me several times in prior positions, but the attempts were deflected with the help of corporate legal staff.

The member appeals process was available and encouraged for all members, including corporate staff. Most of these requests were for referrals or procedures that were obviously outside the terms and limitations of the health care plan. The answer was always the same, "We cannot make an arbitrary and capricious exception to the contract for a dependent of an executive. If you want to make the excluded service a benefit for all workers in that company, please have our legal department draw up an addendum to the benefit plan, and have the compliance department get a sign-off by the state regulators." In a small number of cases, this was done.

For managed care contracts, the claims department could not release the benefit payment without authorization by the utilization review department. Once information is keyed in, it cannot be changed, but additional information and determinations may be added. Someone with security clearance could log on to any case and approve authorization for the service. All the archived dialog screens would be secure, providing an electronic trail of who, what, when and how decisions were made. An audit could show the numbers of approvals and denials by each specific employee.

Of course, many people complain when a service is denied. The appeals process assures that these decisions are reviewed. No one complains when a request is authorized. Would an audit show benefit determinations were being altered without evidence of an appeal process, outside the policies and procedures of MetLife? Would such an audit even be considered? These were questions I did not want to ask, but they nagged at me. Still, when I got back to Miami, I returned to *driving the desk.*

Shortly before Dr. Duvie left MetLife with his wardrobe of empty suits, our Regional Medical Director, Dr. Otto Delupe, interviewed the staff, Dr. Kay Serah and me. Once Dr. Duvie left, the office was split in two. Dr. Kay Serah and Nurse Hatchet would administer the HMO products. I was promoted to the Director of Managed Indemnity and Preferred Provider Organization (MIPPO) products, managing a staff of 30 professionals. I was very grateful to be back in the medical management stovepipe. I initiated a TQM educational effort and management style, which resulted in a significant improvement in employee morale.

Within a week of the management change post Dr. Duvie, Dr. Barrelmaker, the medical director for the AvMed Miami office, contacted me regarding the open assistant medical director position. The Santa Fe Corporation located in Gainesville, Florida, owned AvMed. AvMed had been started by a Miami physician originally doing physicals for the aviation industry, hence the name. It had evolved into a very well run HMO in major Florida metropolitan areas.

We got together for lunch, and he explained the history of AvMed and the duties of the Assistant Medical Director. Over the prior year, AvMed had recruited several of the nurses from MetLife who had recommended me for the position. We hit it off very well, but he understood that my present position with MetLife, if not inspiring, was very comfortable. We discussed my interest in *his* job, concluding that if the corporation ever kicked him upstairs, he should give me a call.

Employment at MetLife, during the late winter and spring of 1993 was somewhat discomforting in its monotony and lack of challenge, even though our team worked very well together. I was managing a group of very professional medical folks. Essentially all the minor, petty, personal conflicts had melted away. The MetLife policies and procedures assured that our medical management, cookie cutter operations ran smoothly. The time demands of managing my team were minimal; I spent most days driving the desk. But I was bored, and the previous several years of watching my back was getting to me.

Only one development during this spring got my attention. Dr. Serah had developed a nurse reviewer report that tracked activity and cost savings. She had used a personal computer and Lotus 1-2-3 spreadsheet software to configure the report. The reports were communicated up the chain of command. The fact that this was going on was not necessarily a professional problem for me, since she managed a separate mini-stovepipe. However, lacking knowledge about personal computing and electronic manipulation of data did make me feel a bit inadequate.

I had a profound theoretical understanding of TQM and statistical process control, but no hands-on training or education with spreadsheet or database programs. I knew how to design a study (e.g., I knew the right questions to ask and the metrics to follow). Reading and understanding reports, formulating solutions and taking appropriate actions was a cakewalk. My fingers were lightening fast on the mainframe dumb terminal keyboard. But I did not know how to bring the numbers together in the kind of spreadsheet report that Dr. Serah had developed.

Becoming a computer program expert user was a necessity. Some of the most powerful people in any organization are those who own, manage, present and distribute data, information and knowledge. I enrolled in a computing class at the local technical night school. This was back in the day of DOS and WYSIWYG (What You See Is What You Get). Graphical user interfaces (GUI) were a few years off.

Although I would not have an immediate, direct, practical business application for this knowledge for several more years, it would help me manage my teams in future positions. My corollary to, "He who has the gold, makes the rules," is, "He who controls the information, owns the gold." After taking several classes, I understood, and had experience with the personal computer tools that control organizations and disseminate information.

Toward the end of April, Dr. Barrelmaker wanted to talk to me about a position at the AvMed Miami office. He was transferring to the Jacksonville AvMed Office, and the medical director position in Miami was opening. My choices were clear.

Continuing with MetLife would provide a steady, safe job, with a very sound company, offering a good chance of slow advancement through the ranks. Nevertheless, the corporate culture at MetLife was essentially grounded in indemnity insurance and at a core level, I did not trust that culture to protect me, should any other difficulties arise. I doubted the course of this juggernaut could ever be turned enough to embrace a corporate culture of Continuous Quality Improvement (CQI), as structured in Health Maintenance Organizations (HMOs). I would never realize the vision working for any large indemnity insurance company.

AvMed, from its inception and at its heart, was an HMO. It may have been smaller and less mature, but these folks were the true believers. We negotiated a reasonable signing bonus and a starting date for early June. I gave my thirty-day notice of resignation to Dr. Otto Delupe at the MetLife Regional Office.

AvMed HMO: June 1993 to March 1995

The change of employment to AvMed brought me a lot closer to home. The AvMed office was located about a mile and a half north and just across US 1, in the arms of the on-and-off ramps of the Palmetto Expressway. The drive was about five minutes on neighborhood roads. I had taken the position of Senior Medical Director in the largest AvMed Health Plan in Florida.

My boss was Bernie Mansheim, the Senior Vice President of Medical Affairs & Chief Medical Officer. He was located upstate at the home office in Gainesville Florida. Bernie had a profound understanding of, and belief in, managed care principles. He had a broad understanding of clinical epidemiology and quality improvement. Bernie was definitely not an empty suit. His job was similar to what mine had been at LNC/EBD. He managed medical operations across the six plan sites within the state of Florida. AvMed was a very young organization and lacked uniformity across operations. To this end, he was in the process of standardizing and expanding medical review criteria. Bernie had a lot to do.

The Medical Management Department of the Miami AvMed Office had been functional for several years, but business operations emulated a physician practicing incident medicine. In other words, in an attempt to achieve consistency of purpose, the medical director and supervisors were practicing crisis management, relying on memory and oral history.

The department consisted of a staff of thirty-five professionals. I discovered there was no policy and procedure manual for the department. Organizational charts showing the reporting structure graphically were out of date. Job descriptions did not describe employees' actual responsibilities. The subscriptions for the resources used to determine medical necessity (Milliman & Robertson[16] and Interqual[17]) were out of date. It appeared job security would not be an issue. There was a lot to do.

The first task was to initiate a CQI management style and develop the first office procedure manual. Workflows were mapped, analyzed and simplified. All job descriptions were reviewed and updated. By including the front line workers in these projects, employee morale and workflow efficiency improved significantly. Subscriptions to medical criteria sets were updated, and a contract for special medical policy assessment with Hayes, Inc. was pursued. The methodology for determining if a requested authorization was for experimental care (developed at EHIC in the late 1980s) was instituted.

I chaired the Quality Activities Committee and directed the development

---

16 See Milliman & Roberson: http://www.milliman.com/home/index. php.

17 See Interqual: http://www.mckesson.com.

and implementation of specific quality studies and activities. These activities ultimately contributed to National Committee for Quality Assurance (NCQA) certification. The credentialing committee was also my responsibility. This committee of health care plan doctors reviewed the applications providers submitted to the plan. Primary source verification of medical education, licensure, certifications and malpractice history were reviewed. Reviewers made a site visit to the applicant's office, which they documented, assuring NCQA standards were met. This amounted to in-depth analysis of physicians and other providers who wanted to deliver health care to AvMed members. The chance of any fraudulent service provider getting through this vetting program was slim to none.

Many health care plans, particularly preferred provider organizations (PPOs), do what I call "yellow pages credentialing." This involves sending applications (with attached fee schedules) to phone book listings of medical care providers. By completing the application and agreeing to the fee schedule, the provider is listed in the network. This approach saves a lot of time, energy and initial network development dollars, but does not necessarily result in a panel of quality providers for the members of the health care plan and does nothing to avert fraud.

Because I believe that virtually all physicians make errors 50 percent of the time due to their universal reliance on global, subjective, memory-based decision-making, we did not follow the "yellow pages" model. We were in the business of attempting to assure that the physicians, and other providers we approved for the network, were a step above mediocrity. (No managed care company is able to build a physician network listing only Albert Schweitzer and Mother Theresa clones.) The quality of care they would provide could result in small, but significant, cost savings by treating patients more appropriately and preventing unnecessary emergency room visits. This selection process is one of the core strategies of managed care organizations.

The HMO could save another 5 or 10 percent of the health care dollar through utilization review techniques that establish medical necessity. Our field nurses made daily rounds to review the level of care delivered to in-patient members and to assure the standards for intensity of service were being met. They worked with our case managers to provide discharge planning and our members received care at home as soon as possible. These quality improvements and cost savings would allow AvMed to offer employers broader benefits at lower costs.

I was the chair of the Member Appeals Committee that made final determinations to uphold or reverse benefit denials, but held only one tie-breaking vote should a deadlock happen. The other committee members were plan providers. A plan member ombudsman held one seat. Although it was often difficult to keep this committee focused on the medical facts, the clinical epidemiology (medical science) and the benefits of the health care plan contract, for the most part, decisions were based on objective criteria.

Emotional decisions by this committee could not be allowed. Before every meeting, I would remind the committee that we were not gathered to play "Queen for a Day," awarding a benefit payment to the person with the saddest story. By definition, such decisions are arbitrary and capricious. An inconsistent, uncontrolled decision-making process would be an unfair claims practice, and strip AvMed of its ERISA protection. The committee was reminded that it was their duty to reverse the denial if there was any doubt the decision under consideration was absolutely correct and defensible. Therefore, benefit denials could be reversed, based on several sound, documentable reasons or for the grey areas where denial may not have been defensible, but never because of an emotional appeal. There was no pressuring of the medical department, or this committee, to bend the proper decision making process by any marketing folks. AvMed was a very ethically managed not-for-profit HMO.

By the end of my first fiscal year, our department had lowered inpatient bed days by 50 per 1000 members. Miami was the largest of the six AvMed plan sites, and we contributed over 90 percent of the total Santa Fe Corporation Health Care Plan retained earnings ("retained earnings" is the not-for-profit phrase for the term "profit.") In the case of AvMed, retained earnings did not go to the pockets of our corporate executives. They were not highly compensated. The mission of the organization was not to make billionaires out of the few, but to provide health care and health care benefits to the many. Retained earnings instead went into research and development, employee training and lower premium rates to allow AvMed to continue to provide quality service for members and providers.

Our efficiency allowed the corporation to provide higher quality health care benefits at a lower cost to our employer groups. The efficiency of the Miami AvMed Medical Management gave me the power to negotiate for additional computer training for our employees, thus realizing Deming Point thirteen: "Institute a vigorous program of education and self improvement."

A local ExecuTrain computer center offered training in personal computer programs. For about $500, a yearlong open enrollment to all training programs was obtained for select employees. Beginner, intermediate and advanced classes were offered for all available business programs. Over the next twelve months, I attended classes in all levels of every program in Microsoft Office and Lotus SmartSuite. AvMed was a great place in a great city. I was proud to be working for this company. Although the vision had to be put away for some time, these were good days.

In 1994, Bernie Mansheim announced he would be leaving AvMed. The company would need a new Chief Medical Officer. As a qualification for the position, "Florida Medical License Preferred" was listed. My medical licenses included Wisconsin and Indiana, but not Florida. The position had little appeal, but I felt all the AvMed remote office medical directors were expected to apply. This position would provide a small increase in salary, but a large separation from life—fulfilling the job duties would mean long, hard hours leaving little time for anything else. Although Gainesville, (the location of the home office) is a University town, it is in located in northern Florida and over an hour away from any deep-water sailing. I knew the vision could never be realized by moving up the ladder at AvMed, but I was beginning to feel that life is too short to continue playing the role of Don Quixote, tilting at windmills.

My professional life as Medical Director of the Miami Plan was very satisfying. The medical management team had documented proof that we were improving quality of care while reducing costs, and this proof of my core beliefs was gratifying. Miami, in spite of the traffic problems, was the best place for us to live. Aside from the occasional hurricane, the weather is beautiful. Biscayne Bay is the premier sailboat-racing venue in the world. The Florida Keys provide a great cruising ground for sailors, and the Bahamas are a short 54-mile sail across the Gulf Stream. Many close friends of ours lived in Miami and the Keys.

Following my interview for the position, I was more relieved than disappointed when senior management brought in an outside, Florida-licensed physician, to fill the position.

Large Case Management

In the fall of 1994, a financial report identified individuals who had received services in excess of one hundred thousand dollars during the previous twelve months. This report was run to find potential cases for our Large Case Managers. One of these cases showed expenses exceeding five hundred thousand dollars. Review of the expenses revealed significant portions of these dollars were being spent on custodial and non-skilled care. These are the types of services provided at home or in a nursing home and include housekeeping, baby-sitting and bathing the custodial patient.

Although these services are covered benefits when a patient enters hospice care, they are excluded by the terms and limitations of health care plans. A nurse was assigned to the case as a Large Case Manager (CM). I worked with her to identify those elements of the services being delivered that were medically necessary, versus those that were custodial and not benefits of the contract. The medical providers involved were contacted and asked to evaluate and update their current treatment plans.

After the health care providers sent in their care plan updates for review, the CM nurse re-assessed the services. The assigned CM nurse would manage all authorizations, maintaining contact with the physicians and skilled care providers delivering medically necessary care. An alert in the member's computer record assured any request would be routed to the special CM. A random utilization review nurse would not be involved in any new requests in order to reduce the chance of benefit authorization for an excluded or limited service.

The CM nurse identified the elements of the provider's care plan that were considered medically necessary and covered benefits, within the terms and limitations of the contract. The primary member, Horace Simpton (this is not his real name), received notice that reimbursement for the excluded custodial care services would be terminated. Simpton filed an appeal regarding the custodial services. The appeal was heard through the standard appeal process and the decision was upheld. Mr. Simpton's lawyer requested a meeting with the executives of the AvMed Health Plan Miami Office. The executives at this meeting affirmed determinations made by the medical management department and upheld by the appeal committee.

This case did not illustrate any attempt to defraud the health care plan. The member's primary and specialty care network providers had developed a comprehensive plan of treatment, which included both skilled medical care and social service support elements. Contracted providers were delivering care, but some of the care simply was not a covered benefit. When this error in payment was discovered, the error was corrected, and payment discontinued. The family was offered training in delivery of care, that was not considered skilled medical service.

The lawyer involved filed no litigation regarding this determination. The decision had been made within the letter of the law and the health care plan contract. There were no grounds for legal action. Having failed to reverse the message and no legal recourse, Mr. Simpton may have decided to kill the messenger.

The Internet had become much more available and widely used for both productive and non-productive purposes. No one had yet coined the terms "cyber-stalker" or "Internet bully," but benefit denial determinations made for the large case described above may have created one of the first. I would soon become the focus of an Internet attack and a central figure in the attempt by state medical licensing boards and medical societies to push back against managed care.

Mr. Simpton registered a complaint with the Florida Board of Medicine that I was practicing medicine without a license. Florida regulations did not require HMO medical directors to have an active Florida license. The job, after all, is about determining benefits for members, not the diagnosis and treatment of patients. My licenses were active in both Wisconsin and Indiana, but not in Florida, where it was not necessary.

Inspector Roman Hunt, an investigator for the Board, came to the AvMed offices to determine if the complaint was valid. Mr. Hunt may have been looking for a facility akin to one of the many sham operators that file fraudulent Medicare claims in Miami. He entered my office and soon realized that he had not entered a medical facility. The HMO business office had no medical equipment. There were no patients waiting to see a practitioner. I was not practicing medicine and the complaint was baseless. I gave him a tour of the AvMed Medical Management floor and explained our workflow and process for making benefit determinations.

Following the tour, I sat with the investigator for a time and explained the benefit determination process. While he was still in my office, a request for authorization of an MRI had come up on my computer. The utilization review nurse had referred the case to me because the member did not meet the medical necessity criteria for the procedure. I made the routine call to the provider in Roman's presence. The provider was not able to take the call that I made to his office and his nurse had no additional information. The primary care physician (PCP) had not seen the patient. This member (with a headache) had called the PCP office to request a referral for an MRI. I believed that the member might actually need to see a doctor to determine if the imaging were necessary. My suggestion to the office nurse: her doctor should consider examining the patient prior to ordering tests, or, if he wanted to send the member to a neurologist, I would put a blanket referral authorization in the computer file.

This routine call helped the investigator understand that the original accusation was baseless and that our business office activities did not constitute the practice of medicine. He stated that he would have to submit his report to the Florida Board of Medicine, but could not predict their determination.

Shortly after this encounter I met the legal counsel and pharmacist from a large HMO based in California. The company had purchased one of the local small HMOs that came with a network of clinics. They needed to restructure the business and medical management operations. We discussed the open position of Chief Medical Officer and Vice President of Medical Affairs. The Miami AvMed medical management operation was in maintenance mode, requiring only a "caretaker" medical director. Taking on this new challenge seemed to be an excellent career move for me.

There would be a significant salary increase and a large signing bonus.

A full disclosure regarding the visit from the licensing board investigator was made to the management team and forwarded to the home office in California. The job offer would come if the Florida Board agreed with the investigator. Several weeks later, my lawyer informed me that the report stating I had not practiced medicine had been submitted by the investigator to the Florida Board. The Board would not be considering the case. This information was delivered to the new health plan executives and the home office in California approved the job offer. Relying on the advice of counsel regarding the Board non-action, I accepted the new position and submitted my resignation to AvMed.

Post AvMed—Crash and Burn: May 1995 to May 1997

Once again, April 1 would be a significant date. It took about a week for me to learn enough about the business and medical operations of this new health plan to realize I should have stayed with AvMed. This new health plan had turned out to have deep structural and possibly state and federal compliance issues. I knew this new job would have me living the ancient Chinese curse, "May you live an interesting life."

The company was located in the Northwest suburbs of Miami. The cross-town, one hour commutes, morning and night in heavy traffic, were the least of my problems. Almost daily for the next three weeks, significant, seemingly insurmountable problems became apparent. I felt like I was in purgatory. It seemed the Florida business unit was operating in a very gray area and that the home office in California may not have understood what they had gotten into. The "Clinic Network" was composed of a large number of small Cuban physician offices that were primarily Medicare and Medicaid billing operations.

A Cuban businessperson owned their computerized electronic billing system. His partner was one of our corporate officers. There were no checks or balances in place, and I felt none would be welcomed. This place made me very, very uncomfortable. Fortunately, Horace, my cyber-stalker, actually came to the rescue. He had been tirelessly lobbying the folks in Tallahassee to do something about the medical director accused of practicing medicine in Miami without a license. The Licensing Board was feeling the pressure.

Three weeks into feeling increasingly uncomfortable in this position, the office of the Board issued a "Cease and Desist Notice." The notice was about the MRI referral process observed by the Board investigator, not about the practice of medicine allegations made by Mr. Horace Simpton. I would find out later that Ms. Bernadette File, a lower-level bureaucrat, issued the notice. The Board never did review the investigator's file, or make any determination as a state regulatory body. In addition, they "lost" the cover letter written by the investigator, which stated, in his opinion, that I was not practicing medicine.

I know I was denied due process of law and habeas corpus. Although a Cease and Desist *Notice* does not carry the weight of a Cease and Desist *Order* (the difference between, "We think you might be a naughty boy" and, "We want you charged with a third degree felony"), the effect on my professional life was the same. I was placed on paid leave for three weeks. A six months' severance package followed. This was my second severance package. I never had a chance to thank my cyber-stalker for getting me out of this very uncomfortable job, even if it was never his intention to help me.

Although I would have liked him to stop right there, he may have felt he had not yet done me enough harm and may have been demanding action by anyone who would listen. The Miami District Attorney's office received the notice. Unfortunately, the issue got into the hands of Bud Uronnar, a third-class Assistant District Attorney. In my opinion, Bud was a low-level prosecutor who did not understand the difference between a *Notice* and an *Order*. He most certainly did not understand the letter of Florida law regarding the practice of medicine.

My lawyer, Xavier Breth called to let me know the Miami District Attorney's Office issued a warrant for my arrest. Practicing medicine without a license is a third degree felony that calls for a heavy fine and jail time. AvMed stepped up to the plate for my defense, paying all legal fees. After about six months, and significant billable hours from a high profile Miami outside counsel, the case finally got into the hands of Mr. Lauren Ordure, a top level, competent prosecutor. It took him very little time to determine no violation of law or regulation had occurred:

- None of the physicians in the network believed I had practiced medicine. They would be adversarial witnesses.
- The State Investigator would be an adversarial witness, having advised the Board he had not observed the practice of medicine.
- The Licensing Board had lost the investigator's cover letter in which he reported I had not practiced medicine.
- The investigator documented that the actions he observed were specifically permitted based on his review of the Florida Statutes and regulations.

It turned out that Ms. Bernadette File, a Board bureaucrat, had issued the notice. There had been no Florida Licensing Board review of the complaint or the evidence. I believe she issued the Cease and Desist Notice based on her lack of understanding of the information gathered at the time the investigator visited the AvMed office. She "lost" the cover letter and failed to understand Florida statutes regarding the practice of medicine. The physicians on the Board never formally reviewed the case, but I believe they were being pressured to "do something." I believe the pressure to do something was coming from Mr. Simpton. The Miami DA's Office dropped the case without prejudice, and expunged the record.

Despite winning the legal battle, I had become the poster boy for the nation-wide crusade by medical societies and medical licensing boards to require state licensure for medical directors working within their borders. The medical licensing boards wanted to take control of the policies and procedures of managed care organizations away from state departments of insurance. Because they were in a different stovepipe of governmental command and control, they were only able to make a lot of thunder and fury.

The political winds against HMOs, fanned by the propaganda of the medical-industrial complex, had grown stronger, but not strong enough to effect the change. The unfounded accusations against me resulted in bringing the struggle for regulatory control of HMO medical management departments into a biased political debate. Some politicians and many yellow journalists were willing to take up flags in this parade. In the end, the medical-industrial complex and the politicians they purchased hobbled managed care. Unnecessary medical care and the cost of paying for this abuse began to skyrocket.

Although this case had illustrated that medical directors should not and typically do not practice medicine, applying medical necessity criteria to determine payment questioned the judgment and authority of the so-called experts. The Emperor did not appreciate being told he was naked. Using standard medical criteria to authorize payment for covered medically necessary health care made organized medicine very uncomfortable. The medical establishment and the rest of the medical-industrial complex had suppressed managed care to maintain power and profits.

I talked to Xavier Breth, my attorney, about taking action against the State Board of Medical Examiners for violating my civil rights, and filing a complaint against the Miami DA's Office for prosecutorial incompetence. Xavier gave me some of the best advice I ever received. He said, "You can't win a pissing contest with the government. The government has an endless supply of piss." There was no point in going after anyone for stalking, filing false reports, or violation of the Ninth Commandment, "Thou shall not bear false witness against thy neighbor."

There was no point in kvetching over this episode. I understood the realities of the situation. There may have been a duty by the Board and the

DA's office to protect my rights and properly investigate the complaint before taking action. AvMed had suffered the financial damages resulting from my legal defense. I had suffered no monetary damages. My income tax filing for the year would show I earned more than the prior year. All that had been assaulted was my reputation and, being a realist, I understand that a medical director's reputation, and a dollar, will get him a cup of coffee at Wal-Mart. I would have to let Karma take care of the bureaucrat, the prosecutor and the stalker.

CHAPTER 7:
The Consulting Phoenix

I had worked in and out of Miami for the previous five years. Miami is the epicenter of Medicare and Medicaid fraud and abuse, but I had limited experience with this indemnity, fee-for-service (FFS) problem. Working within managed care organizations, credentialing, provider contracting, peer review, utilization management, case management and quality improvement processes kept fraud to an absolute minimum.

My last three weeks of full-time employment in 1996 at a company with minimal checks and balances, had opened a window with a view into the dark side of the medical-industrial complex. Extrapolation of the potentials for abuse to completely uncontrolled standard FFS Medicare and Medicaid provided an instantaneous understanding of how billions of dollars are wasted in these programs. As Senator Everett Dirksen famously never said, "A billion here, a billion there, and pretty soon you're talking about real money."[18]

The First Big New Jersey Consulting Gig: 1996

During 1996 and 1997, I completed two big consulting gigs and had hip replacement surgery. An old friend and co-worker from LNC/EBD, David Willis, asked me to assist with answering a Medicare Request for Proposal (RFP). Medicare wanted to determine if managed care processes would improve outcomes and reduce costs for their dialysis patients, a special class of very high cost, service-intense subset of enrollees. A dedicated dialysis

---

18 Senator Dirksen is often attributed with this quote, but his Center says he never actually said it (see http://www.dirksencenter.org/print_emd_billionhere.htm, retrieved on December 27, 2010).

center nurse would do comprehensive coordination and management of all medical services for Medicare patients with end stage renal disease (ESRD).

People with ESRD are placed on Social Security Disability making them eligible for Medicare. With this particular RFP, Medicare was seeking agencies to develop four demonstration projects that integrated managed care with the treatment of ESRD. One of the key elements required in the Medicare RFP was the central role of a Case Management Nurse. The CM nurse coordinates the delivery of care and support services. The clients were being treated at an ESRD clinic, managed by Dr. Royal Payne Diaz, a nephrologist (kidney doctor), and Bill M. Moore Memorial, the associated hospital. The hospital was a kidney transplant center and, as you would expect, was paying for the consultation.

David had put together a small team of consultants for this project. He was the lead consultant and project manager. Sherm Aungst, one of David's network development lieutenants at LNC/EBD, was also brought on board. The RFP required submission of a complete plan for an all-inclusive network of medical service providers, medical management protocols and claims processing. This meant our team had to develop a "virtual" HMO.

If Medicare selected our client for the demonstration project, we could pull the trigger and develop the program in the real world. If it happened, the three of us could have been leading an innovative population management entity. The consult lasted from late summer through early fall of 1996. David and Sherm worked on the business, finance and network elements of the RFP. I developed the quality improvement program, workflow charts, policy and procedure manual, and the job descriptions for all members of the ESRD team. We produced an excellent work product that was dead-on in meeting the requirements of the Medicare RFP. Then, Dr. Diaz and Mr. Adam Illion, the hospital administration in charge of the project, decided to make some modifications before submitting the document to Medicare.

Neither the hospital administrator nor the nephrologist had any appreciation for, or understanding of, managed care principles. They never understood that the role of the case manager was to facilitate better care, not to inspect and report problems with the doctor or facility. I would not say the nephrologist had an ego the size of New Jersey—New Jersey is too small. He and the hospital administrator modified the document so it was no longer recognizable as a managed care response to the Medicare RFP. I believe the physician may not have been able to embrace managed care principles or to share patient care responsibilities with a case management nurse. The key element of the Medicare HMO demonstration project was active participation of the case management nurse to assure all bases were covered, criteria met and costs under control.

The consultant team was paid handsomely for the elegant work product we produced—that the provider and hospital administration subsequently extensively modified. Dr. Diaz and Mr. Illion did not understand the concept, did not respond properly to the Medicare request, and did not get the contract for the demonstration project. Medicare ultimately rejected their response to the RFP. I expect Mr. Illion explained the cost and failure to secure the demonstration project to the hospital board by saying, "We should have gotten better consultants."

Too-Long Delayed Hip Surgery

I put my paid time off to good use. The hip I had destroyed during a high impact aerobics executive fitness program while at EHIC was finally replaced in September. This experience would reinforce my views on our medical delivery system, as I was fortunate to survive the procedure. The system failed even though the *right thing* was ordered. The system failed because the people involved did not do the *thing right*. I was lucky to be a strong patient prior to surgery.

Prior to surgery at South Miami Hospital, I had two units of blood drawn and placed in storage for possible use during my procedure. Hip replacements were fairly bloody affairs back then, and this precaution was the *right thing* to do. The blood bank tapped off two units of blood, spun them down to pack the red cells, and then gave back my serum (it looks sort of like chicken soup draining back in). The packed cells were sent to the hospital for cold storage until the procedure. They were supposed to be available if needed. Unfortunately, I needed this blood, but it was not available. Somehow, the blood bank or South Miami Hospital had "lost" my blood.

Following surgery, the lab test showed I had lost one-third of my red blood cells. This would have been excellent health care for the 1700s, when bleeding the patient was a common practice. It took several days for me to be able to stand for more than three seconds without passing out. My rehabilitation took a little longer than the "average length of stay," for the procedure because I was not able to get the transfusion of my own blood when needed, and was strong enough to spend the extra time letting my bone marrow make them rather than get a transfusion of someone else's blood. I hope my two units of packed cells were put to good use.

Short Consulting Gigs

After my recovery and rehabilitation following surgery, I secured several consulting gigs with managed care organizations to prepare them for the

National Committee for Quality Assurance (NCQA) required certification. From June 1996 to March 1997, my clients included purchasers, MCOs, disease state management organizations, insurance companies, pharmaceutical manufacturers, and health care providers. My past training and work experience allowed me to focus on assessment of compliance, quality improvement, UR, CM, discharge planning, formulary development, provider credentialing and MCO provider network management. I assessed data resources and made recommendations for compliance with the Healthcare Effectiveness Data Information Set (HEDIS) reporting requirements.

The presidential election of 1996 between Bill Clinton, running for re-election, and Bob Dole, running to put America into reverse gear, resulted in a substantial defeat for the GOP in both the popular vote and the Electoral College. President Clinton summed up the Dole campaign when he said, "We do not need to build a bridge to the past; we need to build a bridge to the future."[19] The Republican Party seemed to be ignoring both the pace of technology advancement and the demographics of the country, while looking backward to a mythical time in America that never really existed. I was a child and teenager during the "good old days," and they weren't nearly as rosy as everyone seemed to say. Because of a war wound, Bob Dole carried a pen to avoid shaking hands. At a time when so many people were using personal computers, this protective device seemed to be a metaphor for the yearning to recreate that mythical past. More disturbing was the rise in power of the religious right, which seemed to fly in the face of the GOP's obsessive references to our Founding Fathers. Our Founders had the great sense to separate Church and State in the Constitution because of the oppression and religious wars that dominated Europe. This ideological shift to the right was alarming in many of its consequences.

Equally as frightening was the Republican-controlled Congress hobbling of managed care. The Republican Congress had scuttled the Clinton Health Care Plan. Universal health care had become very important to me personally. Since my six-month severance package and health care benefits had run out in December of 1996 I had intimate familiarity with the angst of being uninsured or underinsured. From January 1997 through April 1997, my wife and I were uninsured and at extreme financial risk should either of us suffer a significant accident or become seriously ill. At this point, I became an "Independent, Centrist Republican," swallowed hard—and voted for Bill Clinton.

---

19 For a full transcript of the speech, see http://www-cgi.cnn.com/ ALLPOLITICS/1996/news/9608/30/clinton.speech/clinton.shtml.

The Second Big New Jersey Consulting Gig: 1997

The second big gig was at a health insurance plan in New Jersey. As was the case with most HMOs at the time, the company was having financial problems, and needed to be "reorganized." Part of the consulting team handled the upper management and financial restructuring. The consultants under contract had lost their managed care medical expert. They called me at the last minute, and my schedule was open.

I was extremely fortunate to have the opportunity to work with Lynda Bluestein, a consultant who worked out of New York. Lynda is perhaps the most knowledgeable, hardest working managed care professional I have ever known. The depth of her knowledge of the business of managed care and the consulting process was only surpassed by her ability to read people and her political sixth sense.

Meetings were held with the medical management staff to document the existing workflows and discuss improvements and simplification. We analyzed workflows and diagramed proposed improvements that we discussed with the employees. The improvement process was taken directly from Dr. Deming's TQM teachings. The new, simplified workflows meant we needed to analyze and rewrite the policy and procedure manual and job descriptions for the medical management department.

We worked many ten- to twelve-hour days, where discussion and analysis followed long meetings. The day would end when we finished writing, editing and printing the documents for the next round of meetings. Although the days were long, the work was interesting and enjoyable. This consult lasted several months. The medical management reorganization plan was completed in February of 1997. I was proud of our work product and very grateful for the opportunity to work with and learn from Lynda Bluestein.

PHP Cariten HMO: April 1997 to June 1998

One of my first gigs in 1996, as I was beginning my consulting career had been with a medium-sized HMO that a hospital system owned in Knoxville, Tennessee. PHP Cariten HMO was facing a state certification review in a matter of months, and had just enough time to prepare to meet the requirements. They were good people, but had not dedicated enough resources to the task. My job was to turn the pieces of the puzzle into the picture of quality. My successful consult led to TennCare recertification for PHP Cariten HMO after their state review process.

Within weeks of the end of the second New Jersey consult, I was called for an interview with PHP Cariten Health Care. They had an opening for

Medical Director of Case Management and Quality Improvement, and remembered how successful the consultation had been. I was offered the position after my second interview. We would keep our home in Miami where our daughter was finishing her PhD in Public Administration at Florida International University. A Residence Inn, once again, served my short-term needs. I moved to Knoxville and started work at Cariten. Kathy would join me several weeks later.

Covenant Health was the premier hospital-based health care delivery system in East Tennessee. To my knowledge, it still is. It owned PHP Cariten HMO, one of the fastest growing, for-profit, managed care organizations in the state of Tennessee. Their managed care HMO products included commercial, Medicare and Medicaid (TennCare) offerings. The Cariten HMO, where I worked, has since been spun off to Humana.

My responsibilities included: 1) pharmacy and formulary management; 2) large case management and policy development; 3) quality improvement and policy development; and 4) the NCQA review preparation effort. Three departments with a total of twenty-three full time employees reported to me. I served as the chairperson of the Quality Improvement Committee, Pharmacy and Therapeutics Committee, and as member of the Appeals and the Cariten Corporate Quality Improvement Committee.

Dr. Rolland Redford, the Vice President of Medical Affairs and Chief Medical Officer, was my boss. Rolland was a southern gentleman doctor from Memphis, Tennessee. Dr. Redford was "born again" and one of the few true Christians I have ever met. He was a trained preacher, having obtained a degree in theology. Although Rolland yearned to be a minister, he and his wife understood the financial realities of life. They had children to raise and educate. He practiced emergency medicine and worked in managed care administration for many years.

Rolland never talked down to anyone; he lived his Christianity. He believed in forgiveness and redemption. He had followed the news reports of my encounters with the Florida regulators and Miami DA, but realized I was not defined by the disinformation on the Web or industry publications. He understood I brought an abundance of skills to the table.

He had also hired Dr. Hirsutus Aurumpton as the Medical Director of Utilization Review. Hirsutus was also a man with a past, who had overcome some major personal and professional problems. Due to his background in utilization review and extensive knowledge of physician practice pattern analysis, Dr. Aurumpton was well suited for his position.

Physician Report Cards at Cariten and Elsewhere

Cariten had a very good database claim processing system. They had purchased an additional software package that used standard query language (SQL) to generate special reports. Hirsutus could "drill down" into the data (or get from the data summary down to some very specific individual points) to generate provider and disease-specific "Episode Grouper Reports" that could show individual data as well as patterns in the data. When a report shows them to be a "high cost" provider, all physicians will say that their patients are sicker and need more medical care than other doctors' patients require.

Episode Grouper adjusted for other conditions and severity of the illness, so apples could be compared to apples, or, rather, doctors could be compared to doctors. The reports spanned an entire episode of illness, hence the name: "Episode Grouper." For example, the total cost and outcome for the treatment of sinusitis could be compared between physicians of like specialties.

There was a wide disparity in treatments and tests orders among physicians, for equivalent outcomes. The "report cards" were developed for sharing with our network physicians. The intent was to inform the practicing physicians how they compared to peers, and to provide information regarding best practices. These reports illustrated the most efficient, lowest cost pathway to achieve the best outcome for the patient.

Our Chief Medical Officer presented Dr. Aurumpton's reports to the Covenant Board of Directors. Rolland experienced a good deal of push-back regarding these reports, especially from the physicians attending the meeting. These fine southern gentlemen physicians may not have received the "report card grades" they felt they deserved. One of the more politically powerful board members, Dr. Reggie Marauder, was particularly incensed. Consequently, the plan to distribute "report cards" and best practice information to our network physicians, using them as part of a methodology to determine quality bonuses, was never mentioned again.

Toward the end of the 1990s, many HMOs had developed such reports. The folks in medical management departments knew where all their contracted network physicians and hospitals ranked, on a scale that ran from "good outcomes, low cost," to "bad outcomes, high cost." For political reasons within the corporation, PHP Cariten HMO was not able to make this private information available to individual physicians. I believe most other organizations had the same problem.

HMOs could not openly publish this information for several business reasons. The HMO had selected these network physicians because of their specialty and location. A physician committee had credentialed them through primary source verification of their certifications and reviewed their malpractice history. If they passed muster and were mediocre or better, they were listed in the HMO Provider Directory and available for member selection. Because of the intensity of credentialing, the average ability to deliver medically necessary care by HMO network physicians would have to be significantly better than the general level of mediocrity for practitioners in the entire community. How would a marketing department turn "We're a little better than average" into a positive campaign? What happens to the practice and cash flow of individual network doctors with report card rankings below average?

The HMO could hardly make physician report cards available to the members and not expect a massive exodus of docs from the plan. Publishing such data would beg the question, "Why did you guys sign up all these bad doctors?" I am sure some politician would criticize the health plan because, "Half your doctors are below average!"

Provider report cards remained confidential. The hospital board blocked distribution of report cards to our network physicians. The report cards were used to develop an internal physician quality bonus methodology. Unfortunately, as with most HMOs of the time, there were never sufficient retained earnings or profits to share with the physicians.

Corporate management provided programs for education and self-improvement, embracing Deming's Point Thirteen. Managers were taught the basics of statistical process control and actively solicited ideas for process improvement from the people working in their units. Continuous Quality Improvement was part of the corporate culture at Cariten. As part of the Covenant Health system, this was to be expected. All hospitals in the US are required to achieve certification by the Joint Commission of Accreditation of Hospitals (JCAH – now called simply the Joint Commission), so robust quality improvement programs are necessary. This corporate culture spilled over into the other health care entities they managed. One of the main facilities, Parkwest Medical Center, only a few miles from the Cariten Health Plan Building complex, hosted operational and educational meetings.

Dr. Aurumpton provided the case management nurses I supervised with disease-specific member reports, identifying high risk, high cost individuals. Each CM nurse was assigned a group of members with similar medical conditions. These nurses became experts on the needs of the members they supported and became very familiar with the physicians and other providers who treated these folks. They were experts in matching the care of the patient to the terms and limitations of the health care plan. The effectiveness of the dollars spent could be maximized for the patient. Working with these professionals and improving the health status of the members they served was an absolute delight.

Despite a Successful Disease Management Program, Red Ink Meant RIF

My position with Cariten would prove to be the most satisfying and productive of my last ten years in administration. In addition to the usual day-to-day medical management business, several special projects were initiated. The development of the disease state management (DSM) program for members with diabetes was the most successful. Management of the morbidly obese was rolled into the diabetes program. An asthma DSM program was initiated.

The main Cariten Heath Plan contract included a clause allowing providers to subcontract out some services. Network service provider sub-units for diabetes and asthma were organized. The morbid obesity program was a natural fit for the diabetes center. Our plan contract allowed the case manager, with my approval, to authorize a "global" fee for all services related to the disease. Managing these diseases not only keeps individuals as healthy as possible for as long as possible, they also keep people out of bankruptcy and keep health care costs from growing out of control.

The diabetes program would eventually enroll over eighty members. Hemoglobin A1c, the metric used to measure diabetes control over time, was reduced from above 9 to below 6. The value, in terms of avoiding human suffering and cost effectiveness, cannot be stressed enough. If a patient with diabetes crashes out of control, the emergency room and hospitalization bills will run tens of thousands of dollars. Most importantly, many people admitted for *ketoacidosis* (high acidity related to a diabetic crash) never leave the hospital alive. In addition, the cost of admission of one diabetic patient in *ketoacidosis* is approximately the equivalent cost of a dozen insulin pumps, which could keep as many diabetic patients healthy for many years.

Similarly, the program that manages a population of patients with asthma will prevent many hospital and ER admissions for respiratory distress and respiratory failure. For such admissions, the mortality rate for patients admitted with respiratory failure approaches 25 percent and the cost is tremendous.

Our team worked very hard to meet quality improvement standards and comply with State of Tennessee directives. As a result, Cariten achieved TennCare (Medicaid) recertification and NCQA certification. The medical management department thereby saved many millions of dollars in unnecessary costs, but all these efforts failed to keep Cariten in the black. TennCare, the state Medicaid Program, failed to adequately fund the system. Unfunded state mandates added to these financial problem. Although he couldn't discuss it at the time, a friend in the Finance Department knew the health plan was bleeding.

Rumor held that the Chief Financial Officer was originally an administrative assistant to a member of the establishment at Covenant. As business operations expanded, her climb up the ladder proceeded rapidly in spite of what seemed to be a lack of formal training or depth of experience in finance. It turned out she may not have been keeping the Board of Directors completely informed about the losses. I do not know if the problem was incompetence, ignorance or just a reluctance to carry bad news to the board, but over a period of weeks the reported loss jumped from $14 million to $18 million. A month later, when the actual loss of $36 million was communicated to the board, the board decided to downsize Cariten.

Unfortunately, many very good people were part of an inevitable reduction in force (RIF). I was one of the executives who were part of the initial wave. We became known as the "Fab Five." The hospital board provided the Chief Marketing Officer, Vice President of Marketing, Vice President of Operations, my friend the Director of Finance and me with six-month severance packages. This was my third severance package. In short order, the Chief Operating Officer Ferris O'Toole and Dr. Redford, Chief Medical Officer, followed us out the door. The Chief Financial Officer was among the first to go as well.

Dr. Aurumpton stayed on board, managing the entire department. Since his salary was well below Rolland's, this made sense. He had obtained his license in the state, and had been generating utilization review reports for management. Once again, the golden rule applied, *"He who has the gold, makes the rules—and—he who controls the information, has the gold."*

Interestingly, Dick Dinglebury immediately hired the Chief Financial Officer back into the Covenant fold after the Cariten RIF. In spite of the massive losses reported in the HMO, the hospital system logged some of their best "retained earnings" years during this period. It makes one wonder if a hospital system has ever owned a managed care health plan that consistently showed black ink. I doubt that these organizations plan to lose some money out of the health care plan pocket while stuffing the facility operations pockets full, but it does seem to work out that way.

My position at Cariten had been cut short. The work had been very enjoyable, and I felt extremely productive. The diabetes DSM program was having remarkable success, but with the Reduction in Force, it probably would not be continued. Short-term tactics would be needed to assure survival of Cariten; a long-term strategy would have to wait for better times.

The RIF, which occurred in June of 1998, was not the worst thing that could have happened to me. My severance pay and medical care benefits would last though the end of the year. I had come to believe that my vision would never be realized, but our retirement plans could be satisfied. Kathy and I had contracted with a boat builder in South Carolina to construct a custom cruising catamaran. When completed, this would be our "live aboard" home for several years. The boat would be fitted out as a floating office, so I could continue consulting from anywhere along the intra-costal waterway. The "keel was laid" and construction of Millennium Dragon began in 1997. Changes in the manufacturing facility location, however, would delay launch until 2000. The second half of 1998, and all of 1999, was open to any possibility. This would be enough time to find another position or consulting gig. The consulting gig would come first.

ESI, Inc., Washington, DC: 1998 to 2002

Several weeks after I left Covenant/Cariten HMO in Knoxville, Tennessee, I received a call from an old friend. He had been working as team leader for a minority-owned company based in Washington, DC. The name of the company was "ESI, Inc." They had a contract with the Center for Medicare and Medicaid Services (CMS) to perform follow-up compliance reviews at designated HMOs. These managed care organizations, for one reason or another, had failed a portion of a site review, or had a sanction that needed further evaluation. Some of these organizations were ordered to develop a CMS corrective action plan.

A team from ESI, headed by a "Lead Physician Reviewer," would perform the site visit and evaluation. They submitted their report to ESI, which was formatted and delivered to CMS. The Lead Physician was considered an independent contractor by ESI, so no benefits were attached to the position. My interview for the open Lead Physician Reviewer Consultant position was successful, and I started work in the fall of 1998.

Through this contract, I would lead several consults per year between 1998 and 2002. The job was a series of gigs at HMOs across the country. The cooperation we experienced from the folks who worked at the health plans was nothing short of amazing. We lead an initial meeting with the CEO, a board member or two and the heads of all the departments involved. We conducted interviews with upper and middle management. We completed analysis of compliance with regulations and corrective action plans. Following three to five days of our evaluation, we conducted a final exit debriefing. The board and CEO attention and concern meant we could expect a high level of cooperation from upper and middle management—that and the fact that if any of these plans did not pass the site visit, they could face fines or could be shut down. The weight of the federal government will get people's attention.

Depending on the parameters of the review, I supervised a team of three to five professionals. Actually, saying I "supervised" them is a bit strong, since each reviewer was also an independent contractor. Every independent contractor would assess the health plan (in his or her area of responsibility) for compliance with the corrective action plan. These were seasoned professionals, all having many years of experience in the industry. They would submit their reports to ESI independently, but I had the responsibility to herd these cats. This was not difficult as all were expert cats that knew their territories very well.

I was directly responsible for evaluation, analysis and timely report submission for the Quality and Utilization Management Sections of the reviews. My duties included promoting positive and productive interaction with the regional and central office review personal and compliance officers of the Centers for Medicare and Medicaid Services (CMS). These federal bureaucrats were consummate professionals. I enjoyed working with them tremendously.

Cornerstone Alliance, Lima, Ohio: March 1999 to April 2000

By the end of the 1990s, email had become an important social and professional networking tool. I notified managed care professionals in my address file regarding my availability for consulting work or an appropriate medical director position. My resume was updated, attached to an email, and sent to my list of managed care executive recruiters. ESI, the minority-owned Washington DC-based CMS contractor, had been keeping me busy. I continued to work for them as an independent contractor until 2002. However, my severance package and medical insurance benefits had ended. In 1999, 38.7 million individuals (or 14 percent of the US population) were not covered by insurance.[20] Additional millions were underinsured. We were among them.

There was an expensive solution to my health insurance problem. In 1985, President Reagan had signed the Consolidated Omnibus Budget Reconciliation Act (COBRA) that would allow me to continue our insurance plan with Cariten. The premium cost over $900.00 per month. Being uninsured and pushing sixty was not a comfortable position, but we were both reasonably healthy. Paying $11,000 for a year of coverage for the one or two routine care medical visits was unreasonable. We purchased a low-cost, defined benefit, high deductable, catastrophic coverage policy. Luckily, we stayed healthy.

---

20 US Bureau of the Census. (2009). Table HIA-1. Health Insurance Coverage Status and Type of Coverage by Sex, Race and Hispanic Origin: 1999 to 2009. Retrieved on December 27, 2010 from http://www.census.gov/hhes/www/hlthins/data/historical/index.html.

Although the executive recruiters were not much help, my networking efforts finally paid off. A former co-worker from my time at LNC/EBD called, letting me know about a medical director position in northern Ohio. She had done some consulting for the organization and recommended me for the position. In March 1999, I secured my last medical director position in the small town of Lima, Ohio.

Lima is located in a large rural farming area in northwest Ohio, along Interstate 75. In 1999, about forty-five thousand residents lived this rust-belt town, which was in decline. Formerly big employers included a small petroleum refinery and an old Ford Motor company plant that built tanks just south of town during WWII. The plant had been converted to Ford engine production after the war. The unionized workers at this plant, like the town, were aging and in decline. The petroleum refinery was directly south of town. The public safety disaster plan called for a lock-down of all businesses in town should a fire or explosion occur there.

There were two competing hospitals in Lima. Lima Memorial Health Center was the smaller of the two. St. Rita's Medical Center was the larger, and is now a level-two trauma center. St. Rita's Hospital sponsored a Physician-Hospital Organization (PHO). The PHO, known as "Cornerstone Alliance, Inc.," had signed a contract with Cigna Insurance, the company that provided medical benefits to the United Auto Workers employed at the Ford plant.

Cigna had transferred risk for all medical services (except for out-of-area emergencies) to the PHO and St. Rita's Medical Center. Cornerstone's Executive Director, Gene Antigua, had come on board after the contract had been signed with Cigna, about a year before I arrived. The prior medical director had been a part-time, semi-retired practicing physician. This kindly, old, well-respected gentleman had apparently treated his position in the PHO as if he were the senior partner in a medical clinic. Benefit authorization requests were approved or denied based on what he believed was appropriate. In actuality, no one denied a benefit payment for any requested care.

His retirement resulted in the open medical director position. Cornerstone needed a managed care medical director. My work began in March. The Executive Director, Gene Antigua, was a managed care professional, with experience in both physician networks and business management. The staff included three registered nurses, a provider relations coordinator, a financial analyst/accountant, a claims coordinator and an administrative assistant. They had been recruited from the local area and St. Rita's Medical Center. While the nurses would report to me, the rest of the staff reported to Gene.

These folks worked well together and, considering there was very little in the way of a written structure in place, performed the necessary managed care functions quite well. A formalized organizational structure had not seemed necessary in the past. Lima was a small town and virtually everyone knew each other. The Cornerstone staff knew the people at the hospital, the network physicians and their private medical office personnel.

Within days, I was able to assess the staff, the business operation and the financial situation. As I suspected, the subscriptions for the criteria and standards manuals had expired. This was an easy fix. A policy and procedure manual would have to be written and job descriptions updated. I had a great deal of resource material in my files so the manuals and job descriptions were completed within weeks. Only a minimal amount of re-writing was necessary to format the information to match Cornerstone's needs. Our small office retained a very informal, friendly atmosphere, but the staff did appreciate having a more formalized structure with regard to business operations and their duties.

The PHO was Born to Lose

Cornerstone Alliance was a financial disaster for St. Rita's. The PHO had essentially two managed care health plan contracts. One was with Cigna, to provide medical services for the United Auto Workers at the Ford plant. The other was with St. Rita's Medical Center, for their employees and dependents. Both these business entities reflected the demographics of Lima. The town was on the decline. There was an exodus of young people, leaving behind a population of older, more medically needy folks.

The Ford plant had a large number of older men who smoked and had heart disease. Due to the age and disease load for this group, the medical loss ratio was upside down. The Ford UAW employees provided a completely new meaning for giving "110 percent." Actually, the medical loss ratio was closer to 120 percent. Cigna appeared to have negotiated a malevolent contract that left St. Rita's Medical Center and Cornerstone Alliance holding the bag. I do not know if the original Cigna negotiators were being consciously predatory, or their underwriters and actuaries simply missed the target. Nevertheless, whatever the reason, the Cigna funding for the medically necessary care delivered to Ford employees was woefully inadequate.

In my opinion, Cigna set the premium rate for the health care plan, low-balled medical reimbursement, took their profit and left the providers holding an empty bag. The best efforts of the medical management team at Cornerstone reduced unnecessary care, but it was never enough to stop the red ink from flowing.

St. Rita's employee health plan was also difficult to manage. St. Rita's was self-insured. This meant the hospital paid for the medical care for employees and their dependents. For any super expensive individual medical expense, they had a reinsurance policy.[21] When I arrived on the scene, the health plan had four strikes against it. The first was that the employees were part of the aging population of Lima. This was not as critical an issue as it was with the Ford plant because overall, fewer employees at the hospital were abusing their bodies, but this demographic did have an adverse effect. The second was that these folks were health care workers. In my experience, health care personnel usually consume more medical services than the lay public. The third, and biggest factor, was that St. Rita's was not unionized, although a national trade union organization was working with some employees in an attempt to establish a union at the hospital. The fourth strike working against us: hospital administration did not want Cornerstone to deny authorization for any unnecessary medical service requested for any employee. The thirteen months I spent in Lima at Cornerstone Alliance were an exercise in frustration, but I knew it was going to be. From the start, the challenges facing the organization were obvious. The wheels were spinning, but nothing was moving.

Cornerstone Medical Director Duties

I lead the Quality Improvement, Credentialing and Utilization Review Committees. A meeting of one of these PHO committees was essentially a "Good Ol' Boy" get together. Lima was a small town; St. Rita's was the big dog. The staff physicians were all members of the same club. Most of the physicians found it difficult to separate St. Rita's hospital staff activities and PHO functions, and these committee meetings reflected the confluence of the work in both places.

There was no "Appeals Committee" structure or protocol. This was not a major issue, since very few official denials ever had to be made. If a request was made for benefit authorization of a service that was clearly not medically necessary, the PHO medical director would discuss the standard criteria with the attending physician, who would generally withdraw the request. Using an informal structure (and authorizing some very questionable medical services) meant that the number of official denials was extremely low. In addition, as the major player in Lima, most medical care was delivered at St. Rita's where all fixed costs of doing business (administrative/professional staff salaries, servicing bonds/loans, facility and equipment cost and maintenance, etc.)

---

21   St. Rita's health care plan was self-funded or self-insured for individual losses up to $100,000 per year. St. Rita's purchased a reinsurance policy to cover individual losses greater than $100,000 per year. "Reinsurance" is insurance for insurance companies. See Wikipedia (http://en.wikipedia.org/wiki/Reinsurance) for a more detailed description of this kind of coverage.

were covered. The marginal cost for St. Rita's to perform any health care service, whether medically necessary or not, was minimal. The only significant cost for St. Rita's would be the professional fee paid to one of their staff physicians.

For example, the facility had an MRI machine and salaried medical staff to operate the equipment. The cost to the facility for doing one more MRI for an employee would be the cost of the paper on the exam table, the electricity to run the machine and the cost of laundering the patient's exam gown. The fee paid their contracted radiologist to read the imaging study had been negotiated. St. Rita's and the radiologist would bill Cornerstone Alliance for the procedure.

I would not call this a shell game, but it was a simple matter of transferring the funds between balance sheets—one balance sheet for St. Rita's, and the other for Cornerstone Alliance, the company they owned. Under these circumstances, any denial of a benefit, for any reason, would result in an upset employee and an upset staff radiologist. With union organizers on the prowl, this just was not going to happen.

Another very important reason their denials were so low stemmed from the fact that Lima was a small town. It is only a slight exaggeration to say that everyone knew everyone else's business. An aberrant physician would soon be identified by his peers and by the town's population. If a doctor were playing patty cake with one of his nurses, his peers and most of the town would know about it. The town was just large enough to offer a selection of physicians to the population, but small enough that a naughty or incompetent doctor would soon be driven out of business.

Small Town Politics

I was not in Miami or Knoxville any more. Although someone might consider Lima provincial, the docs were truly nice guys, with a strong Midwestern work ethic. They delivered a reasonably conservative style of practice, and, by any measure, provided good medical care. This was the brand of medicine I had practiced on the South Side of Milwaukee. Global subjective memory-based decision making was universally operative, but the physicians on the St. Rita's staff could definitely be considered good doctors.

As Medical Director of Cornerstone, failure to organize and make operational an effective diabetes disease state management program was my biggest disappointment. There were major political and regulatory issues that blocked this effort. For provincial political reasons, any community health improvement effort had to be sponsored by both hospitals. One such community-based program, a joint effort initiated and operated out of a small office complex south of St. Rita's Medical Center, provided diabetes education.

The existing program consisted of one nurse and one part-time dietitian. They conducted what I call an "inject the orange and send a post card" program. Patients referred to this center practiced on an orange to learn the technique to inject insulin. At regular intervals, the center sent a post card to participating patients reminding them to see their doctor. Such superficial programs satisfied the requirements of the regulators and NCQA, but could have minimal, probably not measurable, improvement in the health status of the patients involved. Getting both hospital administrations to agree on any improvements to the program would be very difficult.

Politics could make a redesign of the program difficult, but fear of federal regulations from the Center for Medicare and Medicaid Services (CMS) made it impossible. Legal counsel for the hospitals gave the opinion that exposure to federal antitrust action was significant because the effort was supported jointly by two competing entities. The lawyers were worried about the antitrust implications of competing institutions getting together to determine the price of diabetic education or testing services. For this reason, the program had to be offered as a free service to the community. The existing community-based nurse and dietitian diabetes center could not be the pathway to a comprehensive disease state management (DSM) program for diabetes.

A board certified endocrinologist, Dr. Kent C. Deforest, had refused to become part of the Cornerstone Alliance network. He was one of the very few tertiary internal medicine specialists in the area specifically educated and trained to diagnose and treat serious "glandular" conditions. Virtually all patients with any abnormality of the pituitary gland, significant thyroid/parathyroid problems, adrenal gland abnormalities (e.g., Addison's disease), or poorly controlled diabetes were referred to him.

We talked with him several times about joining the network and about the possibility of establishing a diabetes disease state management program in Lima. He would be the logical choice for the Medical Director position. Setting up such a program would provide Cornerstone opportunities for creative contracting through large case management (LCM). The health care contract had a $500 limit for durable medical equipment. This contract limitation put an insulin pump (at about $7,000) out of reach for most people.

If a diabetes DSM Program similar to the entity established at PHP Cariten HMO were established, all inclusive fees for various levels of diabetic services would follow. The individual diabetes goods and services within each increasing level of complexity would be bundled together and the case manager could authorize a monthly management fee without violating the terms and limitations of the contract. For example, the standard contract could limit durable medical equipment to a $500 expense. An insulin pump could improve control but would require the patient to pay several thousand dollars out of pocket to purchase the machine. A diabetes DSM program could bundle the pump with all other associated goods and services in the highest level of care. The physician directing the diabetes center could negotiate a monthly management fee for each patient enrolled in the program with the health care plan medical director. The health plan medical director would authorize payment of the fee to the diabetes center for a particular level of care. The plan would no longer micromanage payment authorization for the individual goods and services subcontracted to the center.

Such an independent Diabetes Disease Management entity would not have to serve only St. Rita's employees and the Ford plant employees managed by Cornerstone. As an independent medical service provider, such a program could be marketed to other insurance companies and managed care organizations; anyone in Lima and the surrounding area who needed the services could get them.

Dr. Kent C. Deforest could not wrap his mind around such a DSM Program. I do not know if he simply did not want to deal with the management issues, or was politically too far to the right to believe any managed care organization promoted health maintenance and preventive care. Whatever the reason, the big picture eluded him. He never joined the Cornerstone physician network, and a diabetes disease state management program never got off the ground in Lima.

Cornerstone Crumbles

The Cigna contract was up for renewal in the fall of 1999, and could not continue as it had been written. St. Rita's had underwritten Cornerstone's red ink for too many years. Obviously, those payers who did not enjoy a discounted fee for service were subsidizing Cigna's profits by paying full price. Cigna was not willing to increase the dollar amount, or percent of premium, they would need to pay Cornerstone to get it into the black. An equitable payment to Cornerstone would increase Cigna's medical loss ratio. The contract was not renewed and, for me, the writing was on the wall.

The future of the PHO was predictable. Gene made a valiant attempt to preserve Cornerstone through marketing our medical management expertise, but Lima was just too small a market. Most businesses will have finalized their budget by the end of the third quarter, or early into the fourth. St. Rita's never published a budget for Cornerstone after the Cigna contract was terminated.

We continued to administer the managed care plan for the Medical Center employees, but I knew my days were numbered.

My last project for Cornerstone and St. Rita's was submission of a comprehensive appeals process policy and procedure manual. I put this together after the hospital administration reversed a denial for a procedure that was clearly not a benefit of the contract. For reasons stated before, such an action exposes the health care plan (in this case, St. Rita's since they were self-insured) to unacceptable risk.

The appeal policy and procedure manual designated, by title and by name, the people who would sit on the committee. Several administrators in upper management at St. Rita's, including the Vice President of Nursing, were included. The corporate counsel was included. As support staff, the hospital medical librarian was included. She would provide the medical research regarding the status of specific medications, testing or treatments. Physician board members were included. The Cornerstone administrative assistant would record the meeting, supplying secretarial support. One patient advocate, selected at random from the plan members, would attend each meeting. During the appeals process, all patient records would be edited to remove any reference to the member or physicians involved, providing complete objectivity for the process.

The manual I wrote offered guidance for proper decision-making procedures, including several example scenarios of proper and improper denial reversals and confirmations. The cover memo to the appeals manual suggested that the hospital employees establish a "sunshine fund" to help pay for services that were not covered by the health care plan. St. Rita's could contribute to the fund, but it would essentially be employee-supported and controlled. A "sunshine committee" would be established to determine who should receive a grant for excluded health care services and how much should be given. This would be the Queen for a Day, Home Makeover, sad-stories-always-make-me-cry committee. It would not be part of the benefit plan.

A copy of the manual and cover letter were delivered to all identified parties in early February of 2000. At the same time, I requested a meeting with St. Rita's Medical Center senior management team to discuss the proposal and get their input. At this point, the Cigna contract was gone, and Cornerstone had no budget for the year. The meeting date, time and place I suggested were put on hold. The end was near, but there was no way of knowing how long St. Rita's would continue supporting the staff at Cornerstone.

On the more upbeat personal level, Millennium Dragon, our cruising catamaran, had been launched and final commissioning was underway. We would be able to move aboard between April and June so the timing of my resignation was important. At the end of February, the budget for Cornerstone was finally published. Cornerstone would be continued, but the Medical Director was reduced to quarter time. The same day I was called into the human resource department and presented with a severance package. They wanted me to continue "on call" for three months, followed by a six-month continuation of salary and benefits. This severance package was my fourth and would carry me through the end of the year 2000. A few other consultations with ESI in Washington DC would provide some extra money into 2002, but essentially, I was retired.

I had not come to Lima to change the world. This job was about medical benefits and to generate some income until I retired. I applied my skills and knowledge to the tasks, but I had no great expectation that anything significant could be accomplished. St. Rita's Medical Center made a reasonable business decision with Cornerstone. The contract negotiated with Cigna, early ineffective medical management and the size of the service area made the outcome predictable.

The people at the Cornerstone office were good folks who knew what they were doing and worked very hard within the confines of the health plan. Hard work was not enough. The politics of medicine and doctor preconceptions about managed care once again stood in the way of developing programs that would improve people's lives. The project was financially doomed from the start due to the contract with Cigna. Another hospital owned-managed health plan had essentially gone under because of financial problems.

Retirement: April 2000 to the Present

Kathy and I left Lima at the end of March and moved aboard our cruising catamaran, *Millennium Dragon*. We lived aboard at a dock at Port Royal Landing Marina in South Carolina until we finished fitting her out. We learned much about the cruising life from the local live-aboard cruisers in that time. Working from the boat, I would complete several more managed care site reviews for ESI through 2002, but I consider this my post-retirement work.

Through my career in managed care administrative medicine, I had gained profound knowledge of why medical care lacks quality and costs so much. I had developed the vision of a future medical care delivery system that would address and resolve these issues. Although some minor skirmishes had resulted in small victories during my career in the managed care industry, all the battles I and others waged, and eventually the war, had been lost. Most famously, President Bill Clinton and First Lady Hillary had made a valiant effort to reform health care, but in the end, politics overcame reason for the larger political arena just as it had been thwarted along the way during my professional life.

Leaving work behind was not difficult. We had been preparing for this transition for thirty years, saving for retirement and investing in our future, which was now upon us. I had spent the previous eight years in simmering frustration because I could find no way to implement the vision. The assault on managed care had continued. The cost of medical care and the lack of quality had not been painful enough for the country to raise a call for reform or change. I had to try to accept the fact that the *vision* was not going to happen, and I should let it go.

I watched the 2000 election with interest from the boat. As a registered Republican, John McCain got my vote in the primary. By the time the election rolled around, we had done a little cruising and seen the plastic trash and tar balls that washed up on the beaches. I became convinced that our country had to address our environmental problems and stop polluting the planet. Al Gore got my vote ultimately because George "W" seemed excessively far right and Gore promised to do something about those tar balls. Al got the majority of votes; "W" won the election. Saving the environment, like health care reform, would have to wait.

During the first three years of retirement, Kathy and I lived aboard the *Dragon* while cruising the intra-coastal waterways, Florida Keys and the Bahamas. My log of our adventures starts with the statement, "You've got to be ready to die." The direct reference is to dropping out and leaving your friends, family and most of the land-locked stuff of modern life behind. Sailing off to the small family islands of the Bahamas, where the phones do not work and the mail boat brings almost fresh fruit and vegetables once or twice a week, requires that you put affairs in order.

During that time, the Taliban blew up the ancient Buddhist statues in the Bamiyan Valley in Afghanistan, George W. Bush and our Republican Congress passed the largest tax cut in history, and Muslim religious extremists attacked the World Trade Center Towers in New York. The invasion of Afghanistan started October 7, 2001. Our cause was just. The world was with America and supported this action. It appeared we could be successful with a minimum loss of life and treasure. Although the Bush tax cuts meant it would have to be financed through credit, the war was expected be limited and short. Our economy was supposed to be strong enough to support the debt. Although the cost of medical care continued to rise, no one seemed interested—the war distracted everyone. Then came the Iraq war, which never seemed to be justified well enough. Moreover, taxes were not increased to cover the cost of waging two wars. The party of fiscal responsibility was not being fiscally responsible. We returned stateside and found a house on a canal with a dock for Millennium Dragon in Punta Gorda Florida.

The efforts of American right wing religious extremists were blurring our constitutional separation of church and state. On July 19, 2006, Bush used his veto power for the first time in his presidency against the Stem Cell Research Enhancement Act. The vetoed bill would have repealed the 1995 Dickey Amendment, which prohibited the use of federal funds for the creation or destruction of human embryos for research purposes. Ultimately, such research has the potential to find a cure for diabetes, Parkinson's disease and a host of other conditions. This Act was an example of how much power the right wing religious fundamentalists had in our government and how effective their war on science had become.

On August 9, 2006, our grandson, Antonio Julian was born. The frustration I had been feeling about the direction the country was taking became unbearable. Our grandson could live eighty or more years, and I feared he would have to live through the "Second Dark Age" right-wing Christian and Islamic religious extremists are attempting to impose on the world. America and the rest of the world seemed to be on the path to perdition.

August 27 2007, was my sixty-fifth birthday, making me eligible for Medicare. Having retired in the year 2000, Kathy and I were *under-* or *uninsured* for about seven years. We had been very lucky to avoid any catastrophic illness. Like all Medicare-covered individuals, we are allowed to select a health plan on a yearly basis. I reviewed all the Medicare offerings available in Charlotte County, Florida, and picked the best plan. My wife and I chose coverage by the Medicare Advantage Humana plan. The HMO Advantage plan is a government (taxpayer) financed public option, administered by Humana, a for-profit corporation with stock traded on the NYSE. The "Purchaser" is the government (we, the people), and the administrator, or "Payer," is Humana. The "Providers" are the local private physicians, facilities, durable equipment suppliers, pharmacies and a Punta Gorda health club in the Humana "Network." Kathy and I were very, very happy with our "government run health care."

Toward the end of 2007 and all of 2008, the housing bubble burst and our financial markets collapsed. By the time of the presidential election, over two-and-a-half million jobs had been lost. The need for a change in direction was almost universally recognized. Candidate Barak Obama offered a message of hope that made sense geo-politically and economically. His position on the wars and on human rights took the moral high ground. He recognized that the reformation of our health care system was necessary. The 2008 election ushered in a Democratic majority in both the House and Senate along with

President Obama. I watched with interest as campaign promises on health care translated into positive accomplishments of governing.

During 2009, I closely followed the Democratic Party's formulation of and attempts to pass so-called "Health Care Reform" by negotiating away much of what could have been effective financing reform. The GOP continued to complain about Democratic Party efforts without publishing a program to address the medical cost problem. Mainstream Republicans have stuck their collective heads in the sand, insisting the American health care system is the best in the world, ignoring all information to the contrary. Republicans attempted to block passage of "Obamacare" using poorly veiled ideological rhetoric, becoming the party of "hell no."

It became clear to me that Democrats do not understand the cause of the health care crisis, and Republicans do not recognize there is a crisis. Our for-profit insurance industry remains focused on producing dividends for shareholders and bonuses for executives. I just could not take it anymore. There was no time left to wait for the world to change. I had to take action and began writing in February 2009. Showing the vision for health care and the path we as a nation must take to achieve it had been an important personal goal. I sincerely hope these efforts are not another exercise in frustration.

Epilogue

As 2010 came to a close, we needed to make a change in our health care plan. Our Medicare Advantage Humana HMO plan notified us they were dropping the Silver Sneakers[22] program (a fun, energizing program that helps older adults take greater control of their health by encouraging physical activity). I doubt that the decision makers at Humana realized Silver Sneakers is much more than a feel-good program that promotes socializing for old folks. Kathy and I had attended exercise classes three times a week and Zumba workouts twice a week for over a year. This health improvement program had produced measureable benefits for both of us. Promoting regular exercise would have similar health improvement benefits for most seniors—and most people in general.

A major secondary benefit that the bean counters who made the recommendation to drop the program may have missed is the reduction in "medical loss ratio"[23] for Humana by promoting health and wellness. This

---

22 For more information about the program, see: http://www.silversneakers. com/

23 "Medical Loss Ratio" is the percent of insurance company premium dollars paid to health care providers for covered medical goods and services.

benefit goes well beyond the obvious improvements for the individual and concomitant lower medical costs. Including a limited membership to an exercise facility attracts a healthier senior population. Healthier seniors have lower health care costs than those with chronic debilitating diseases. Promoting the Silver Sneakers is a legal way for Medicare Advantage administrators to select a healthier, lower-cost population. Dropping the program is a good way to let healthy seniors know they are not valued. For-profit insurance companies are often unable to see beyond the quarterly report to shareholders to understand how these less tangible benefits can truly affect the bottom line.

Humana may have had other Medicare plans that covered Silver Sneakers. It didn't matter. Their business decision was not in my best interest or in the best interest of folks enrolled in their HMO plan. I had to send a message to Humana, no matter how small or insignificant it might be. Kathy and I switched our coverage to the American Association of Retired Persons (AARP) United Health Care Secure Horizons[24] plan so that the Silver Sneakers wellness program would be covered.

I doubt that the bean counters at United Health Care have a significantly different mindset than the bean counters at Humana. I am sure neither group spend much time looking past the next quarterly report. However, by switching Medicare Advantage plans from Humana to AARP United for 2011, Kathy and I were able to keep the same physician and continued membership in the Silver Sneakers program. And we are now very happy with this new government-financed Medicare Advantage health care plan as administered by AARP United.

---

24 See https://www.securehorizons.com/

CHAPTER 8:
Doing the Right Thing and the Thing Right to Improve the Health Care System

I expected to write this manuscript in five or six months. It has taken much longer and been significantly more difficult than anticipated. The manuscript has evolved into two books. This first book, *Discovering the Cause and Cure for America's Health Care Crisis,* is my memoir. It is presented in a way that shows how my experiences have shaped my own understanding of the issues. I wrote it to help everyone in America understand our current system and what we need to do to fix our problems. The second book, *Creative Design for Health Care Reform,* offers a more technical analysis of our present health care system and presents a business plan for resolving our cost and quality problems.

In 2009, the U.S. National Health Expenditure (NHE) grew to $2.5 trillion, or $8,086 per person, accounting for 17.6 percent of the nation's Gross Domestic Product (GDP).[25] The World Health Organization (WHO) ranked the United States number thirty-seventh in the world for health care in 2000, the last year for which these statistics are available.[26] We can all agree that we

---

25 Centers for Medicare & Medicaid Services. "National Health Expenditure (NHE) Fact Sheet." Retrieved on January 18, 2011 from http://www.cms.gov/NationalHealthExpendData/25_NHE_Fact_Sheet.asp#TopOfPage.

26 World Health Organization. (2000). "The World Health Report 2000—Health Systems: Improving Performance. Downloaded on January 27, 2011 from http://www.who.int/whr/2000/en/index.html.

need to do something to improve our health care system. Just what we need to do is the subject of this and the next book.

As 2010 ends and I write these last lines, the American economy has gotten worse. The rising unemployment numbers driven by our deteriorating economy pushed the voters to the right, allowing the GOP and Tea Party to take control of the House of Representatives. I believe the newly elected members of the House and Senate are about to gain first-hand experience regarding the huge difference between promises made during a political campaign and the potential for positive accomplishments while governing.

It will take several years before Americans will know if the actions of Congress during the first two years of the Obama Administration will stand. If they do, it will take several years to determine if they make a difference. In the meantime, our domestic economy remains in peril. I am hopeful that the new Congress will govern by making informed, intelligent decisions. Obstructing programs and sitting on the sidelines are not viable options. Too much is at stake. The decisions our elected officials make during the next several years will determine if we are entering a new golden age or the beginning of the decline and fall of America.

As a sailor, I don't need a meteorologist to tell me when I'm in a hurricane. As a retired small businessman, medical professional and insurance executive, I don't need an economist to confirm that the world economy is in the toilet. As of this writing, Greece and Ireland are bankrupt and Spain is on the slippery slope. The only difference I can see between the 1930s and today is that the regulations and social safety net put in place after the Great Depression have covered up and softened the profound nature of our present economic crisis— we were flirting with a national average of about 10 percent at the worst in 2009[27] rather than an overall 25 percent unemployment rate in the peak of the Great Depression in 1933.[28] However, the widespread economic decline for many middle- and working-class families has been equally devastating, and many groups (such as lower skilled and minority groups in larger urban areas) have seen Depression-like unemployment figures over 20 percent.[29] These

---

See "Annex Table 1 Health system attainment and performance in all Member States, ranked by eight measures, estimates for 1997"

27 Bureau of Labor Statistics, www.bls.gov.

28 VanGiezen, Robert, and Albert E. Schwenk. (originally posted fall 2001). "Compensation from before World War I through the Great Depression." Bureau of Labor Statistics. Retrieved on January 18, 2011 from http://www.bls.gov/opub/cwc/cm20030124ar03p1.htm.

29 Filion, Kai. (2010, January 14). "Downcast Unemployment Forecast— Targeted Job Creation Policies Necessary to Offset Grim Projections."

days of job scarcity, foreclosure, global unrest, and natural disasters may soon become known as the "Second Great Depression"—some are already calling it the "Great Recession"; many people worldwide are hoping and praying that better times are right around the corner.

WWII pulled us out of the Great Depression. Although that War put us deeply in debt, it put people to work. It had also destroyed the productivity of the rest of the industrialized world. America was able to pay the war debt because we were the only industrialized country left standing and our products were in high demand. We were also the breadbasket for the rest of the world. There was no competition.

Our situation today is very different. We are now in two small, limited wars that are simply consuming lives and treasure. China and India are becoming industrial super powers, producing the things the world wants and needs. Our balance of trade is negative. Both unemployment and the cost of labor are high. A major reason for our crippled economy, and the one domestic policy we can control to some extent, is the tremendous cost of our health care delivery system. Getting control will save American business, and will improve the health of our economy as well.

Why We Need to Reform the System: Health Care for Everyone will Save American Business and Keep People Healthy

The cost of labor is one of the main reasons that American business is no longer competitive in this global economy. The American economy will not recover until domestic businesses are able to lower the cost of labor and get folks back to work without negatively impacting take-home wages and salary. The cost of health care is a significant percentage of the cost of labor, and skyrocketing health care insurance premiums must become more affordable; health care costs should not break the back of business or the employee.

For example, recent studies indicate a low rate of compliance regarding the purchase and completion of the course of prescribed drug therapy.[30] People forget or don't like to take their medication, or the treatment plan is complicated, or the patient is unable to comply for other reasons. However, a very important part of this problem is the cost of required medication and

---

Economic Policy Institute. Retrieved on January 27, 2011 from http://www.epi.org/publications/entry/ib270/.

30   Lars Osterberg, M.D., and Terrence Blaschke, M.D. "Adherence to Medication." N Engl J Med 2005; 353:487-497

the state of the American economy. Simply put, many cannot afford to buy the pills they need to keep themselves healthy.

To reduce the cost of health care benefits, our government must reform both the medical benefit financing system and the health care delivery system. Unfortunately, Congress has focused on regulating for-profit insurance companies rather than reforming the overall American health care system. Band-aid politics, even when it comes in the form of 2,000-plus pages, will not be enough to improve employers' ability to maintain their competitiveness in this global economy.

According to the Congressional Budget Office (CBO), financial administration could consume up to 26 percent, or $647 billion of the $2.5 trillion spent on health care in America every year.[31] In his book *Prescription for Real Healthcare Reform* Howard Dean stated the cost of health care administration is 29 percent.[32] Real financial administration reform could save more than half (about $331 billion per year),[33] but requires that Congress and the President restructure the process of transferring wealth from the workforce to the providers of medical goods and services. The processes within our for-profit health care administrative services industry as described herein are the product of present laws and regulations that govern the insurance industry. Congress must change the law to change the health care financing system.

Two structural drivers are responsible for the excessive cost of financial administration. The first is that the current system requires employers to be the primary means of access to private health care funding for individuals. This is a problem because: 1) not all Americans have access to jobs that provide benefits; 2) through cost shifting by providers, those with benefits pay for the care of those without benefits; 3) access to funding through relatively small groups of employees requires underwriting to manage risk. Underwriters help maintain insurance profits by rating techniques including pre-existing condition limitations, up-rating and denial of coverage. Our present system of accessing health care financing through employment produces what some folks call invisible "golden handcuffs." Health care financing is not portable. Access to health care binds the worker to the employer, and throws people without those handcuffs to the wolves.

---

31 See: http://www.naifa.org/advocacy/health/documents/Comparing_
    HealthCare_Admin_Costs.pdf Table 3

32 Howard Dean. (2009) Prescription for Real Healthcare Reform, Chelsea
    Green Publishing. Vermont pg xvii

33 See: http://www.naifa.org/advocacy/health/documents/Comparing_
    HealthCare_Admin_Costs.pdf Table 2

The second cost driver is the methodology of transferring health care dollars from the worker to the provider by for-profit, risk-managing indemnity insurance corporations. This is a problem because: 1) for-profit publically owned corporations manage business to maximize short-term shareholder profit, not quality care for patients; 2) the executives take egregiously excessive salaries and bonuses for producing shareholder profits; 3) selling many unique insurance benefit plans to many relatively small employer groups requires a huge, expensive marketing and sales force; and 4) managing the risk of insuring relatively small employer groups to assure profitability for shareholders requires a large staff of professional medical underwriters.

Insurance companies currently limit the loss (control their expenses) of doing business through underwriting techniques. Risk managing, for-profit indemnity insurance companies use the medical histories of employees and the expense history of employers to estimate medical costs for a group of people. Underwriting techniques manage risk based on averages, and can mean outright denial of coverage or increased premium prices with pre-existing condition exclusions. Not all Americans have access to the health care they need or deserve because the underwriting system does not include a large enough base of people to spread the risk of any one catastrophic condition within any particular group coverage plan.

Effective reform could virtually eliminate fraud and abuse, which flourishes in some areas due to certain problems in the system that we can fix. I assert that abuse of the system takes the form of ordering and delivering unnecessary medical goods and services, whether knowingly or in error. Fraud is a criminal act that includes billing for medical goods and services never delivered, usually for patients never seen. Fraudulent billing has been estimated to cost $60 billion each year.[34] Health Maintenance Organizations (HMOs) offer the most effective structure to eliminate fraud by managing provider networks. The HMO subjects the provider to extensive credentialing (vetting) and a site inspection prior to signing a contract. HMOs do not have any phantom providers of medical goods or services.

Two additional realities of the current system that deal with fraud and abuse are important to understand when considering finding cost savings in the system. First, the cost of administrative functions, and therefore the medical loss ratio (cost of health care), depends on the wealth transfer (financing) model. Standard Medicare shovels money out the door through third party

---

34 National Health Care Anti-Fraud Association. "Consumer Info & Action." Retrieved on January 18, 2011 from http://www.nhcaa.org/eweb/DynamicPage.aspx?webcode=anti_fraud_resource_centr&wpscode=ConsumerAndActionInfo.

administrative claims processing. Standard Medicare administrative cost can be as low as 2 or 3 percent, but without well-funded fraud detection and prosecution, $60 billion in fraud per year is tolerated.[35] The administrative cost for HMOs and MCOs is relatively high because an investment is made in processes that eliminate fraud and reduce unnecessary medical care. For-profit insurance companies have administrative costs somewhere in between, depending on the size of executive bonuses and shareholder dividends. Without understanding the total cost (health care services plus administration) for each model, it is impossible to legislate a fair medical loss ratio (percent of dollars spent on health care). One size does not fit all. Congress and the President must recognize that the administrative costs to manage provider networks, standardize criteria for care and improve quality pay a huge return on investment in fraud elimination, quality improvement and reduction in unnecessary medical goods and services.

I understand the politics and public relations need to focus on the percentage of dollars spent on health care (a mandated minimum medical loss ratio), but this provision of the Affordable Care Act puts the cart before the horse. It secures the profits of indemnity insurance companies while weakening quality improvement and cost containment efforts of HMOs and MCOs. Congress and the President must understand that legislating a one size fits all percentage of the health insurance dollar that goes toward administration underfunds the quality and cost containment efforts MCOs can make and locks in profits for indemnity risk managing insurance companies.

The second feature that encourages excessive cost, fraud and abuse is our fee-for-service (FFS) reimbursement methodology. The physician's income is based on the number of goods, services and procedures they provide, not the number of patients they keep healthy. Cash flow drives the quantity, not the quality, of the medical goods and services provided. FFS reimbursement invites physicians, consciously and unconsciously, to abuse the system. The doctor needs some skin in the game (they must share in the financial risk) so that conservative decisions and quality outcomes are rewarded.

Financial methodologies that address this flaw in the primary care, gatekeeper model include techniques such as global fees, case management fees and capitation. Specialists at the secondary and tertiary levels could continue a modified FFS reimbursement methodology, because the gatekeeper model would assure reimbursement for only medically necessary referrals

---

35 National Health Care Anti-Fraud Association. "Consumer Info & Action." Retrieved on January 18, 2011 from http://www.nhcaa.org/eweb/DynamicPage.aspx?webcode=anti_fraud_resource_centr&wpscode=ConsumerAndActionInfo.

and medical care. The modifications to FFS reimbursement now under consideration include payments based on value, results, performance and outcomes. Assuming claims payers apply reliable metrics to determine the quality of care delivered, these payment schemes align reimbursement with cost effective, quality care.

Both political parties have recognized there is a great deal of fraud in American health care, and have projected the dollar savings we could achieve through reform, such as savings on the $60 billion in fraud discussed above. However, following the successful war that many politicians waged against Managed Care Organizations (MCOs) during the 1990s, neither political party is willing to accept the reality that the managed care techniques involving contracting with providers and managing health care networks eliminate most fraudulent billing. Likewise, many folks deny the ability of HMO techniques of utilization management, case management, disease state management and quality improvement to minimize abuse by denying funding for unnecessary and inappropriate medical care. I've seen it work throughout my career in administrative medicine. These techniques lower the cost curve while facilitating quality care and better outcomes for the patient, but they have higher administrative costs. Once the President and Congress understand these realities, we may get the health care system that Americans deserve, but clearly, they do not yet have the knowledge they need to take appropriate legislative action.

Reforming health care financing could save the nation $373 billion every year in health care administration cost. These health care financing savings could flow directly to employers (reducing the cost of labor), and to taxpayers, who support all government-administered health care benefits. However, political and media attention paid to the role played by for-profit, risk managing indemnity insurance companies has ignored the 900-pound gorilla in the room. Congress, the American people and our physicians will not reform our health care system until they understand that our health care cost and quality crises are "just what the doctor ordered." Literally.

A doctor's order is required to get reimbursement for covered health care. Studies published in the Dartmouth Atlas has documented that 40 percent of the physician directed health care dollar is wasted on inappropriate, ineffective or harmful health care goods and services.[36] This empirical evidence supports my considerable experience: up to half the dollars spent on medical goods

---

36 See, for example, <u>Regional and Racial Variation in Primary Care and the Quality of Care Among Medicare Beneficiaries</u> (http://www. dartmouthatlas.org/downloads/reports/Primary_care_report_090910. pdf)

and services are simply not necessary. Doing the math, real reform of health care delivery could the country save over $700 billion per year, which could directly go toward more productive business investment.

The Real Solution: Fixing the Dysfunctional Decision-Making Process

Above, I've addressed the administrative issues and managed care techniques that must be used to make the health care system more efficient and increase positive patient outcomes. I've outlined why we must make these changes. This section discusses how to fix our dysfunctional health care system through addressing the medical community's decision-making process. Three major points must take priority in this respect.

1. Physicians and physician educators must recognize they are at the center of our health care crisis. Our health care crisis will continue to escalate until physicians recognize use of our dysfunctional memory based decision-making process is the cause. Physicians will make a quantum leap in quality improvement and cost reduction when they fully integrate electronic health records (EHRs) and knowledge couplers with their real time practice of medicine.

The entire $2.5 trillion cost of the American medical industrial complex is a direct result of how physicians think, make decisions and get paid. The major driver of excessive cost and abuse is the result of the flawed memory-based decision-making process physicians primarily use to diagnose health issues and determine treatment plans. This failure is the result of the limitations of the human mind, which is no fault of the physician.

The real problem is that physicians and medical educators fail to recognize this limitation and the central role it plays in the inability of the American health care system to deliver cost effective, quality health care. Until physicians and educators understand and take ownership of this failure, effective tools to manage our mental limitations will not be developed or implemented. In essence, the epiphanies I describe in earlier chapters are about recognizing this failure. My vision is centered on understanding the potential role technology can play to help us improve the decision-making process. The future of American health care depends on whether you will join me in pushing the powers that be to recognize the need to develop and use these technological and managerial tools.

I hope that I've convinced you that physician real time application of the EHR and intelligent medical decision support tools is the best way to assure the delivery of quality, medically necessary health care.

2. We must create a foundation of problem oriented electronic medical

records (POEMRs) to replace our current paper-based, and electronic health record (EHR) source-oriented system.

The source oriented electronic health records (EHRs) now in production simply facilitate appointment scheduling and maximize FFS billing (in other words, they improve cash flow, but not patient care). In the past, if an EHR was part of the software package it reproduced the architecture of paper charts to automate the record filing system. The software vendors using this source-oriented EHR filing architecture did not maximize the potential of the new electronic tools to document the physician's decision-making process. Medical decision support tools, in particular medical artificial intelligence, are not present or not fully integrated with the EHR. The future American health care system must be built on the foundation of the problem oriented electronic medical record (POEMR). Refinement, further development and implementation of POEMR with fully integrated medical decision support tools in medical offices across America is the most important step to take toward establishing quality, cost effective medical care for all citizens. This is the essence of technology with a human touch.

3. Short term, government regulations will address cost and quality issues until these electronic tools are built and implemented. We must establish reliable metrics to generate provider and facility "report cards" to give consumer-patients the full information they need to make decisions about where to seek quality health care.

A short-term improvement in the delivery of quality care will be made when the health care consumer—the patient—can read "report cards" that use reliable metrics to assess providers and facilities. The concept of making provider report cards public may run counter to my Deming quality improvement philosophy but it is a short-term strategy for reaching a more meaningful end. Perhaps airing dirty laundry will incentivize folks to prevent soiling their linen and to use washing machines that are more efficient.

Discussions about consumer-based health care and controlling costs through competition are meaningless and a waste of time if report cards do not become a reality. Public records are necessary to separate the good (or at least, mediocre) over the truly bad providers and facilities so that the consumer-patient can make more informed decisions about their care. It would make a small town like in Lima Ohio of the entire nation, where letting the light in keeps everyone more honest. Report cards will drive early adaption of POEMRs with integrated intelligent decision support tools, as this is the only way to achieve the quantum leap toward improved quality and cost reduction.

Scenarios similar to the one Uncle Allen faced need not be repeated if individuals have this information. If my experience with the PHP Cariten

HMO (described in Chapter Seven) is a reliable indicator, it will take an act of Congress before consumers see these health care report cards, and that act is not likely to come soon without public pressure.

What Should Have Happened during the 111th Legislative Session, and What Actually Happened

To fix our economy, Congress must address the structural problems driving the American administrative cost and health care quality crises and embrace managed care techniques. The $1.25 trillion (half our $2.5 trillion yearly health care cost) in potential annual savings for American business and taxpayers will remain potential savings until Congress and the President move toward real health care reform. Until this happens, the American economy will continue to circle the drain and close in on the economic death spiral. The rest of the world's industrialized democracies have pushed the health care financing envelope and achieved quality care for their citizens at a much lower cost, mainly by taking steps toward universal health care financing systems. Their provider reimbursement models foster more conservative medical practices, while producing measurably better outcomes for their citizens. Health care in America remains mired in a swamp of expensive mediocrity. Fixing this must be one of our top priorities as a nation, and it is certainly something we can do if we roll up our sleeves and get to work.

The simplest, most elegant reform that Congress could adopt to address both financial administration issues is to offer reform that provides universal, single-payer funding, administered by private, not-for-profit claims processing organizations. Many liberal news commentators and some politicians have discussed using the name "Medicare for Everyone" or "Medicare Part E" to describe this reform effort toward universal coverage. Medicare Part E would disconnect patient access to health care funds from employment. Instead, taxes withheld at the "community rate" would take the place of inflated for-profit insurance company premium dollars. Medicare Part E would have provided each American a completely portable individual health care policy paid from the risk pool of over 300 million citizens, regardless of their employment situation—if they change employers or become unemployed or self employed, every American would have been assured access to health care funding. Medicare Part E also would have placed each American citizen in the largest self-funded risk pool in the world, eliminating the need for underwriting. Rather than additional mandated insurance regulation, America would have taken the first real steps toward health care reform.

Conservatives condemn universal health insurance as "Socialized Medicine." Taxpayer-funded private claims processing is not socialized medicine. Socialized medicine would follow a system like that of Great Britain, where most physicians are employees of the government. Our present taxpayer-supported Medicare funding mechanism uses private claims processing, insurance companies and MCOs to pay private medical providers for health care services for covered individuals. It is actually a form of public-private partnership; a solution to public financing that is in very good standing with capitalist ideals.

Reform would simply expand the present system to all Americans. The self-funded, self-insured model (universal taxpayer-supported claims administration) eliminates the need for and cost of underwriting. Marketing and sales costs are cut to the bone. Eliminating financial risk management would dramatically reduce administrative costs and most of the reward associated with managing risk. All companies managing the transfer of wealth from the workers to the providers would come to function like not-for-profit organizations. Administration by not-for-profit claims processing organizations eliminates the need to show profits to shareholders and limits egregious executive salaries and bonuses.

The Obama administration proposed the "Medicare Part E" model described above in its original discussions of health care reform. However, Congress rejected this model very early in the legislative process. Conservatives called it "socialized medicine" and the public believed them.

Some Democrats proposed the "Public Option" to preserve the right to purchase for-profit risk managing indemnity insurance privately. This proposal allowed access to Medicare for those unable to acquire coverage from an insurance company willing to assume the individual's financial risk. A public option to purchase Medicare Part E for all Americans could save billions of dollars in health care cost and put pressure on for-profit insurance companies to set competitive prices. Congress rejected this model later in the legislative process.

Congress eventually cobbled together a 2000-plus page rendition of insurance regulations commonly referred to as "Obamacare" that would have made Rube Goldberg proud. Although the Affordable Care Act (ACA) that President Obama signed into law may be the nostril of the camel in the tent, it is not health care reform and will do little to help American Business in time to shorten our Great Recession. ACA imposed insurance regulations that stipulate the minimum percentage of premium dollars allocated to health care (medical loss ratio). This regulation is counterproductive to control fraud and abuse and to reduce the cost of employee benefits and labor. By requiring a portion of the uninsured to purchase insurance, the ACA will assure additional customers for insurance companies and profits for their shareholders.

Keep in mind that the application of quality outcome measurement requires information mined from the databases generated through the use of computerized patient medical records. The ACA promotes implementation of electronic health records (EHRs), quality metrics and documentation of meaningful use[37] (documentation that use of the EHR produces cost effective, quality health care).

To date, attempts to tame our 900-pound gorilla by managed care innovators, the President and the Congress have failed because they focus on the results of the decisions, and do not take the decision-making process into account. Financial incentives and disincentives can move the physician's practice patterns in a more conservative, cost effective direction, but financial incentives are only a part of the solution.

Politicians Require an Infusion of Common Sense and Moderation

Both of our major political parties have been blinded by issues that cloud their ability to solve our health care crisis—and some have lead the efforts to distract the public from seeing the problem clearly or understanding the simplest solutions. The stampede of the GOP to the extreme right triggered by populism and religious conservatism run amuck will ultimately lead to the marginalization of the Republican Party. The GOP must connect the dots between business competitiveness, the cost of labor and the cost of health care. Republicans must transition from obsessive adherence to a far right dogma to a more centrist ideology, and truly become "compassionate conservatives." The Democratic Party must recognize that medically necessary health care for all is not simply a basic American right fought on an ideological battlefield. Focusing on the progressive politics of the left to justify such a socially conscious entitlement program will not carry the day. The issue of universal health care transcends the politics of the left and right. Health care reform is the essential ingredient to the health of American businesses, the economy and the public. The majority of Americans want our political parties to work together to put our country back on track, and it is their responsibility to give the people they represent their best efforts in this important work.

I believe that revitalizing the American economy involves three foundations: 1) Rebuilding the middle class through progressive tax policies for businesses and individuals; 2) Supporting education and scientific research with significant public and private investments; and 3) Reforming the American health care system. *Discovering the Cause and the Cure for the*

---

37   See U.S. Health and Human Services web page: http://healthit.hhs.gov

American Health Care Crisis addresses only the third of these pillars, but the three are linked. America cannot afford to let any one crumble or our economy will not be able to avoid the economic death spiral. Rigid adherence to the dogmas of the far political right or left will scuttle any practical solution to our problems. Congress cannot pass laws based on personal misinterpretations of selected passages from the Constitution or Christian Bible that pander to a small, active minority while suppressing the rights of all Americans. We must maintain absolute separation of Church and State. The majority of Americans do not want to create a theocracy, like Iran, by simply substituting the Bible for the Koran. The GOP and the Democratic Party would do well to remember Senator Everett Dirksen once said: "I am a man of fixed and unbending principles, the first of which is to be flexible at all times."[38]

The not-so-silent majority will not tolerate the repeal of Social Security or Medicare, and a quiet majority supports Congressional efforts toward health care reform. To be effective, governance must balance liberal and conservative views to level the playing field for all Americans. James Madison, one of the Founding Fathers warned against the power that vocal "factions" (interest groups, in today's lingo) seek to establish their own interests, especially if they deny rights to others outside the faction or are contrary to the interests of the community at large.[39] His words ring especially true about health care in America today.

The Republican and Democratic Parties can save themselves and the economy by working together to focus on improving America's ability to conduct business. The clear and present danger to American business and our larger economy is the cost of health care. The solution to this problem, and the only path that will lead to economic recovery, is reforming the American medical-industrial complex. I want to see the Republican Party leading that parade, not dragged along by it, kicking and screaming all the way into the future. This book offers Americans of all stripes some issues to consider as we struggle forward in reforming the health care system. Walter Cronkite once said that America's health care system was neither healthy, caring, nor a system. I am working to do the right thing and do the thing right to make this change, and I hope you will join me.

---

38 Quoted in Kenneth H. Ashworth (2001). *Caught Between the Dog and the Fireplug, or, How to Survive Public Service*, p. 11.

39 Madison, James (under the pseudonym "Publius"). (1787, November 23). "The Federalist No. 10." Retrieved on December 27, 2010 from http://www.constitution.org/fed/federa10.htm.

Appendix

CQI Applied to the American Health Care System

My vision combines most of Dr. W. Edwards Deming's quality improvement methods with most of Dr. Lawrence L. Weed's philosophy of and approach to the provider side of our health care system, modified through my tendency to always question authority and look for answers. This section briefly describes the original work of these two great men and my modifications and explanations for adaption of Dr. Deming's concepts with Dr. Weed's influence to our medical-industrial complex.

I became aware of W. Edwards Deming during the late 1980s when I was sent for training to learn his Continuous Quality Improvement (CQI) management method, Fourteen Points and Seven Deadly Diseases of American business. Dr. Deming's 1986 book, *Out of the Crisis,*[40] is a very difficult read requiring a deep knowledge of business. That same year, Mary Walton collaborated with Dr. Deming to write *The Deming Management Method,*[41] which presented the same concepts for the layperson. Dr. Deming's book was reprinted in 2000.

Dr. Lawrence L. Weed determined that medical errors were primarily the result of the physician's flawed decision-making process. In effect, the physician is at the center of both the flawed process and delivery of the service. His focus was on the problems in medical education, medical records and medical decision making. Decisions made using "global subjective memory-based" intuition rather than scientific evidence based on standards of clinical epidemiology, produce an error rate approaching 50 percent. His early book, *Medical Records, Medical Education, and Patient Care: The Problem-Oriented*

---

40 Deming, W. Edwards. (1986). *Out of the Crisis.* Cambridge, MA: MIT Press.

41 Walton, Mary and Deming, W. Edwards. (1986). *The Deming Management Method.* NY: The Berkley Publishing Group.

Record as a Basic Tool, [42] proposed a radical change from source-oriented to problem-oriented medical records and from incident-based charting entries to notes following the S.O.A.P. (subjective, objective, appraisal, plans) principle. Each patient problem required a structured plan consisting of: 1) Goal of treatment; 2) Basis for the problem statement; 3) Status of the problem; 4) Disability from the problem; 5) Parameters to follow (both symptomatic and objective) and treatments; 6) Investigation to rule out what diagnoses and by what means; and 7) Possible complications. [43]

Dr. Weed developed personal computerized patient medical records and medical decision support to shift the physician decision-making process to base it on clinic evidence rather than memory. His computer programs supported his new medical records model. Dr. Weed understood the difference between doing the "right thing" and doing the "thing right." He wrote *Knowledge Coupling: New Premises and New Tools for Medical Care and Education,* [44] a book about computers in health care, in 1991.

I realized that many of Deming's concepts had direct application to our health care system. With profound knowledge of CQI came an epiphany, and CQI became one pillar of the foundation for my vision. My contacts with Dr. Weed, the father of the Problem Oriented Electronic Medical Record (POEMR), and his concepts about medical education and decision making, became another pillar. My experience in private practice and administrative medicine formed the third pillar. The blend of my education, training, life experience and contacts with these two intellectual giants resulted in the formulation of my vision of the future American health care system.

Transformation of Health Care Through Application of the Fourteen Points

Deming's Fourteen Points and Seven Deadly Diseases focused on improving the quality of manufactured goods and services through improving workflow processes and following production with statistical analysis. He believed that most errors were directly related to the process, and rarely resulted from an individual worker's mistake. Flawed workflow processes produce

---

42 Weed, Lawrence L.. (1970, c1971). *Medical Records, Medical Education, and Patient Care: The Problem-Oriented Record as a Basic Tool.* Chicago: Press of Case Western Reserve University.

43 Weed, Lawrence L.. (1991). *Knowledge Coupling: New Premises and New Tools for Medical Care and Education.* Springer-Verlag, N.Y. Page 21

44 Weed, Lawrence L.. (1991). *Knowledge Coupling: New Premises and New Tools for Medical Care and Education.* Springer-Verlag, N.Y.

predictable error rates. Dr. Deming understood that quality improvement depended on improving the process. Below, his Fourteen Points are described, as adapted to the field of health care, with a brief explanation of why this is important or how it could work.

1. Create constancy of purpose toward improvement of the quality of medical goods and services, with the aim to become competitive and to stay in business.

    Point One is analogous to the First Commandment for business. It focuses upper management of all entities in the medical-industrial complex on quality. These folks may be hospital administrators, insurance company executives, medical chiefs of staff, HMO medical directors or clinic medical directors.

2. Adopt a new philosophy. We are in a new depressed economic age and the age of managed health care. Western management must awaken to the challenge, must learn their responsibilities and must lead for change.

    Upper management must acquire profound knowledge of quality improvement and lead the parade toward the future rather than be dragged along kicking and screaming.

3. Cease dependence on error identification and report cards to achieve quality. Eliminate the need for error identification on a mass basis by building quality into the delivery of medical goods and services in the first place.

    Point Three is not applicable to the health care setting; our present quality assurance methodology is at odds with it, and as I argue in this volume, we need publically available report cards to allow the consumer-patients to have more of the information they need to make a good decision about where to go to get good health care. Publically available report cards showing the error rates and outcomes of facilities and providers are required in the short and medium term to assure competitive pressure on cost and quality. In the future, the problem oriented electronic medical record and intelligent medical decision support tools used in real time will assure the "right thing" is done for the patient, making report cards less meaningful.

4. End the practice of awarding provider network contracts on the basis of fee for service (FFS) cost. Instead, minimize total medical

cost through elimination of unnecessary health care. Reduce the number of providers for any one specialty service (limit the provider network) on the basis of established physician to patient ratios, health care outcomes, and a long-term relationship of loyalty and trust.

> *Point Four addresses both the upward cost pressure of FFS reimbursement and the direct relationship between the number of specialty physicians and the cost for specialty care in defined areas as documented by the Dartmouth Atlas. Capitalistic supply verses demand economics do not work in our medical-industrial complex. More surgery is done in areas with an oversupply of surgeons. FFS reimbursement pays doctors more if they deliver more medical goods and services. Primary care physicians must be converted from FFS reimbursement to global management fees or capitation to orient them toward managing the health of their population of patients. Specialty care physicians must be converted from FFS reimbursement to a value-based fee system. The ratio of doctors (by specialty) to patients must be balanced across the country so health care services are available in presently underserved areas using network contracting, reimbursement and licensing pressures.*

5. Constantly and forever improve the American health care system to improve quality and productivity, and thus constantly decrease costs.

> *Improving the quality of the American health care system requires the efforts of everyone working in our medical-industrial complex. The term "quality" is poorly understood by the public and many physicians. Quality medical goods and services are appropriate (medically necessary), effective (produce good outcomes), efficient (save time and money), and accessible (available to everyone who needs it; in other words, quality care is universal health care and care available in underserved areas).*

6. Institute training on the job.

> *Dr. Deming believed every individual should spend 10 percent of their work time in training. New computer systems, including problem-oriented electronic medical records and intelligent decision support tools require significant training of both medical staff and physicians. Training has extraordinary high value as the quality of care in our American health care system and hundreds of billions of dollars in cost savings hang in the balance. It must be prioritized*

for all levels of the workforce; we can not afford to let training be the first item to cut from the budget.

7.   Institute leadership (see Point 12). The aim of leadership should be to help people, and machines and gadgets to do a better job. Leadership of management in government, medical education, insurance companies and HMOs is in need of overhaul, as well as leadership of production workers (doctors).

Leaders have a duty to gain profound knowledge of quality improvement and a deep understanding of the technology and systems needed to deliver quality care to all Americans. Leaders have a further duty to assure the technology is advanced, tools developed and systems made available to health care decision makers—then get out of their way.

8.   Drive out fear, so that everyone may work effectively within the medical-industrial complex.

The vast majority of errors are the result of faults in the system or process. To reduce errors and improve quality, the folks working in the trenches must not work in fear of being blamed for system errors. They must be valued for their input regarding system and process improvement. Applying Point Eight to the false premise that fear of malpractice drives overutilization must be avoided. Injuries to patients (malpractice) and excessive ordering of medically unnecessary services are both the result of the failure of the memory-based decision-making process. The so-called "malpractice crisis" is an example of our medical professionals playing the blame game when they should be looking in the mirror for the answer. Malpractice reform may just shield our physicians from reality, introduce hubris into the equation and result in more injuries to patients.

9.   Break down barriers between administrators, primary care physicians and medical specialists. People in medical research, information systems, medical management, delivery of care and claims processing must work as a team to foresee problems that may be encountered in the communication and the delivery of medical goods and services.

Point Nine gets to the heart of population and disease state management where a coordinated team of medical professionals cares for a group of patients with complex, costly medical needs.

Managed Care Organizations (MCOs) and Health Maintenance Organizations (HMOs) broaden application of this concept to a broader segment of the population through standard case management (CM) activities. This model, advanced to the extreme, describes how health care should function. In this model, the primary care provider (PCP) manages and coordinates all patient care. It is essentially a version of the gatekeeper HMO model I worked in back in 1985.

10. Eliminate slogans, exhortations and targets for the work force (e.g., number of in-patient days per thousand patients) asking for new levels of productivity.
    Dr. Deming realized that the system and process determined the productivity and error rate. Pushing workers to improve quality, increase production and cut cost without providing new tools and improvements in the systems and processes is an exercise in futility. It also creates fear and frustration in the minds of the workers.

11a. Eliminate work standards (i.e., quotas—patients/hour, claims/hour, days/thousand insureds, etc.) in health care offices/facilities, insurance company or HMO production areas. Substitute leadership.
    The focus on meeting arbitrary work standards detracts from the attention that leader must pay to continuous improvement of the system and processes. The system determines the result of any measurement. Leadership must focus the attention of all managers and workers in any enterprise on continuous quality improvement.

11b. Eliminate management by objective. Eliminate management by numbers. Eliminate numerical goals. Substitute leadership.
    Most American business enterprises manage using short-term objectives. The numbers must look good for each quarterly report. This focus on the short term is one of the reasons for our present economic problems. Management by short-term goals and objectives is also a major cause of our health care cost and quality crises. Instead, we have to look to our leaders to guide us towards long-term goals and objectives.

12. Remove barriers that rob people in financial administrative and health care management, and health care providers of their right to pride in their workmanship. The responsibility of all health care

system workers must be changed from sheer numbers to quality. This means complete abolishment of the annual or merit rating system and of management by objective (or management by numbers).

Deming believed employers must compensate workers relative to their value to the enterprise. If the enterprise did well, the workers should do well. He believed merit ratings, management by objective and management by the numbers caused system problems. People will do what they must to maximize their personal merit rating even if the efficiency of the systems and processes are undermined. The job of the managers in our medical-industrial complex is to facilitate system and process improvement and remove barriers that prevent providers from delivering quality medical goods and services.

13. Institute a vigorous program of education and self-improvement.

Dr. Deming felt on-the-job training in the process was important (see Point 6), but he also believed any educational or self improvement program, no matter how unrelated to the worker's job, would ultimately result in benefits to the business enterprise. Workers must be supported in their efforts to educate and improve themselves. However, the educational system must be carefully considered. Dr. Weed believed our medical education system has failed by producing memory-based so-called "experts" who deliver a high level of unnecessary medical goods and services, thereby abusing the system, whether intentionally or due to the inefficiency of the memory-based training. The goal of medical education and training must be to improve problem-solving capability and learn to use new electronic medical records and intelligent decision support tools.

14. Put everybody in the health care system to work to accomplish this transformation. Transforming the system to lead to better quality of health care is everybody's job.

Continuous quality improvement must become part of the culture for every organization and everyone working in our medical-industrial complex. Our health care system needs small groups of trainers and facilitators to help executives, managers and workers to understand quality improvement concepts so they may properly apply this knowledge, but quality improvement is everyone's job. If we delegate the responsibility for quality improvement to a committee, organization or regulator, we all fail.

215

Diseases that Stand in The Way of The Transformation

Deming's Seven Deadly Diseases discuss the obstacles that will arise as we seek to make this important transformation. Below, his Seven Deadly Diseases are described, as adapted to the field of health care, including my comments.

1. **Lack of constancy of purpose.** We must plan health care innovation and medical services to improve quality and reduce costs to keep the company, facility and provider in business.

   The focus of leadership and all people working in the medical-industrial complex must be on improving the quality of medical goods and services. Goals and mission statements should be developed to keep everyone on track and periodic review to ensure that we have not strayed from these goals can help the leadership keep quality improvement in all things the primary focus of the entire workforce.

2. **Emphasis on short-term profits.** We must discourage short-term thinking (just the opposite from constancy of purpose to stay in business), fed by fear of unfriendly takeover and by push from bankers, owners and shareholders for dividends.

   A reality check is needed for this deadly disease. The American public and our elected officials must resolve several moral and ethical questions:

   1) Is health care a right or a privilege?

   2) Must workers continue to access health care financing through employment?

   3) Should the federal government (the universal tax payer) purchase health care claims processing directly (Medicare for everyone)?

   4) Should for-profit or not-for-profit claims processing operations manage transfer of funds from the worker to the provider?

   Deadly Disease Two dissolves away if access to health care financing is uncoupled from employment, premiums to risk managing for-profit insurance companies are traded for withholding tax and the federal government finances Medicare for everyone.

3. **Use of personnel evaluation systems.** We must be careful about applying a personnel review system, or evaluation of performance, merit rating, annual review, or annual appraisal, by whatever name,

for people in management, the effects of which are devastating. Management by objective, on a "go, no-go" basis, without a method for accomplishment of the objective, is the same thing by another name. Labeling this management by fear would be more accurate.

Management by fear without a method for accomplishment must be eliminated.

4. **Mobility of management.** We must make sure that good managers stay with the company and avoid "job hopping" to the extent possible.

    Dr. Deming noted that job mobility ("job hopping") for top executives was a problem because continuity and consistency of purpose can be easily lost. Job mobility also impacts the company because they lose the experience and institutional knowledge that these employees bring to the table, and they lose the investment they have made in training the individual. Good employees are valuable assets in many ways, and a good business principle is to retain their best workers.

5. **Use of visible figures only.** Management must use "visible figures" with little or no consideration of figures that are unknown or unknowable.

    Measurement is key to improving quality. You can't manage what you don't measure, and you can't improve what you can't manage. Finding the right measurements will lead to improvements in quality. However, it is important to use "visible" measurements—those that are easily understandable and measureable. For example: What is the average blood sugar value among the patients participating in a diabetes DSM program versus patients receiving general care in the community? Some important concepts are difficult to measure, or unknowable. For example: How do you know if the physician is a good human being? How do you measure bedside manner?

6. **Excessive medical costs.** We must be aware of the constraints that the medical benefits package puts on the employer and control those costs wherever possible.

    Dr. Deming recognized medical cost as a major deadly disease but had no answer for solving the problem. He overvalued expert opinion and organizational memory. Although he was the father of continuous quality improvement, he did not understand that our cost crisis is directly related to our quality crisis. How could he know? He lacked profound knowledge of our health care system. His statistical process control methods were modeled for improving the things produced in a manufacturing plant. He had never met Dr. Lawrence L. Weed and didn't understand that the process failure in the health care system is memory-based decision making by our physicians. Central to our quality problem and the enemy of clinical epidemiology and evidence-based medicine are overvalued expert opinion and organizational memory. This Deadly Disease is one of the reasons I wrote this book. More information about it can be found throughout the volume.

7. **Excessive costs of liability.** We must do the right thing and do the thing right not only because it is good work ethic and will produce better outcomes for patients, but as a result, will also reduce the number of cases that have a chance to go to court.

The cost of liability and warrantee are very high for business. Focus on total quality improvement lessens the risks, but business must have some protection from predatory lawsuits. The issue of malpractice in medical care is a paper tiger. The cost is a minimal part of the health care dollar, but has been portrayed as a major problem affecting health care reform efforts. Physicians who order excessive, medically unnecessary care because they fear malpractice litigation is overblown and an example of physicians playing the blame game. Malpractice reform will only have a positive effect when our government ties protection and immunity to decisions made using patient electronic medical records and intelligent decision support tools.

Although Deming's Fourteen Points and Seven Deadly Diseases focused on improving the quality of manufactured goods and services, as illustrated above, they can easily be applied to the health care system. Improving workflow processes and following production with statistical analysis helps identify errors that are directly related to the process and produce predictable error rates. Dr. Deming understood that quality improvement depended on improving the process. The Fourteen Points and Seven Deadly Diseases, as described above, provide a terrific blueprint to help us begin our journey to a better health care system that can provide quality care for all Americans.

Glossary

ACO	Accountable Care Organization—An organization of health care providers that agrees to be accountable for the quality, cost, and overall care of Medicare beneficiaries who are enrolled in the traditional fee-for-service Medicare program.
Administrator	A company offering health insurance products and claims paying services (a.k.a., Payor, payer).
ASO	Administrative Services Only—A claims processing company usually doing business with self-insured employers to administer a benefit plan. They do not manage financial risk.
Beneficiary	A person designated by an indemnity insurance company as eligible to receive insurance benefits.
Benefit	Amount payable by the insurance company to a beneficiary, when the insured suffers a loss covered by the policy.
Benefit Design	The selection of services, providers, and beneficiary obligations that create the scope of coverage.
Capitation	The payment of a per head amount for a defined package of benefits. The purchaser pays a specific dollar amount per member per month to providers for which they deliver specific services, to a defined population.
CM	Case Management—A system for assessing, referring, and following up on patients in order to ensure the provision of comprehensive and continuous service and the coordination of reimbursement for care.

CME	Continuing Medical Education
Community Rate	Health insurance premiums based on a community wide rather than group-specific basis. HMOs are required to community rate.
Cost Shifting	The technique of setting rates artificially higher than actual costs to recover unreimbursed costs from the uninsured, underinsured, other payers and government.
CPT	Current Procedural Terminology—A standardized medical coding scheme developed by the AMA listing thousands of medical services—updated annually.
CQI	Continuous Quality Improvement—A customer focused initiative requiring that processes be analyzed, measured, improved and evaluated on an ongoing basis.
Credentialing	The process of reviewing a provider's academic, clinical and professional ability to determine if criteria for network contracting are met.
Defensive Medicine	The physician practices with the goal of reducing the risk of a liability claim (e.g., performing unnecessary diagnostic tests).
Dependent	A dependent is a person related to the primary insured. They may be a spouse or child. The insurance company or MCO defines coverage.
DSM(1)	Disease State Management—A defined program of medical management for a high cost, complex disease structured as a partnership between the patient, the medical care providers and financial administrator initiated to improve outcome.
DSM(2)	Diagnostic and Statistical Manual of Mental Disorders—A standardized coding scheme developed by American Psychiatric Association listing mental health conditions and their diagnosis.
EHR	Electronic Health Record—Patient medical charts kept in computer files, a requirement of HIPAA.

EMR	Electronic Medical Record—Patient medical charts kept in computer files. Synonymous with EHR.
Encounter Data	An office visit where services are provided and a claim is filed, but no fee is paid. The data is used for financial management of capitated providers.
Enrollee	Individuals covered by MCOs (HMOs & PPOs) are referred to as enrollees, members or beneficiaries.
ESRD	End Stage Renal Disease—Kidney failure requiring ongoing treatment. Persons with ESRD are eligible for Medicare.
Epistemology	A theory of the nature and grounds of knowledge.
Exclusions	Clauses in an insurance contract that deny coverage for select individuals, locations, or risks (e.g., experimental care exclusion).
Experience Rating	The insurance company evaluates the risk of an individual or group by reviewing the applicant's health care cost.
Fee Schedule	A list of fees for all CPT codes used by a health care plan or the government to reimburse providers on a fee-for-service basis.
FFS	Fee-for-Service—Payment methodology whereby Providers are paid individual fees for each service documented and billed. May be paid by the patient or the Payor (e.g., insurance company, TPA, ASO, HMO, etc.).
Formulary, Drug	A list of prescription drugs covered by an insurance plan or HMO. Reimbursement varies for generic, legend (name brand) and off formulary prescription drugs.
Gatekeeper	A PCP responsible for providing or coordinating all aspects of a patient's medical care and pre-authorizing specialty care referrals.

Health Care Delivery System	A combination of employer groups, providers, government agencies and insurance companies working together to deliver health care to a population.
Health Plan	Various types of MCOs. The term is used to differentiate managed care plans from indemnity insurance companies.
HHS	US Department of Health and Human Services.
HIPAA	Health Insurance Portability and Accountability Act—Required providers to comply with specific regulations regarding medical records and billing.
HMO	Health Maintenance Organization—A business that offers prepaid, comprehensive health coverage for both hospital and physician services using a network of health care providers using a fixed structure or capitated rates.
HMO, Group Model	Usually a HMO that assumes risk and processes claims but contracts with large clinics (outsources health care) to provide medical services to members. The groups may be capitated for their services.
HMO, Staff Model	Usually a vertically integrated organization that assumes financial risk, processes claims and provides health care to its members, usually using salaried physicians.
Hospice	A program that is licensed to provide supportive care of the terminally ill.
IPA	Independent Practice Association—A loose confederation of small groups or independent solo practitioners banded together to contract with an HMO to provide health care to its members. The IPA may be capitated or individually paid FFS.
ICD 9-CM	International Classification of Disease—A standardized medical coding scheme for categories of disease developed by World Health Organization listing thousands of conditions.

Indemnity Insurance	Insurance providing a defined level of reimbursement for medical expenses, without regard to the actual medical expenses. The patient pays the difference between billed and covered medical cost.
Indemnity Insurance Company	Usually a for-profit risk managing claims processing company that pays defined fees for medical services delivered to an insured. They generally have no direct relationship with providers.
Insurance Reform	Legislating Changes to insurance companies' practices that prevent high risk/cost consumers from obtaining health care coverage. Mandating increased risk/cost results in increased insurance premiums.
Insured	The insured is the primary person eligible for insurance coverage under a FFS indemnity insurance company. Also know as, a "Member" or "Enrollee" in various health care plans.
Invasive Procedures	Medical procedures that involve the introduction of a medical device below the level of the skin.
Knowledge, Declarative	That which is known by past training or experience (example: knowing a list of phone numbers).
Knowledge, Procedural	Knowing how to do something that is known (example: knowing how to look up a phone number).
Living Will	A legal document generated prior to illness by an individual to guide providers on the desired medical care when the individual is unable to communicate his or her own wishes.
LOC	Level of Care—An assessment of the intensity of service and severity of illness is used by UR nurses in a MCO to determine medical necessity for payment authorization.
LOS	Length of Stay—MCO UR nurses use average length of stay tables by condition to determine payment for the initial number of hospital days preauthorized.

Loss Ratio	The ratio of the all claims made against an insurance policy divided by the total premiums taken in. Loss ratios are used to indicate the portion of benefits returned to policyholders.
MBS	Medicare Benefit Structure. The minimum benefits defined by Congress that all Medicare "Insurance" plans must cover.
MCO	Managed Care Organization—The combination of financial risk management and health care delivery with application of medical standards to determine quality and reimbursement.
Medical Loss Ratio	The total medical expenses/total revenue received.
Medical Underwriting	The determination of the individual's or group's health cost risk. Individuals or groups may have their past experience or medical histories reviewed by an underwriter prior to coverage approval.
Medically Necessary Care	The delivery of a service or treatment is appropriate and justified when the patient's medical parameters meet nationally recognized standards and criteria.
Medicare RBRVS	Federally mandated Medicare "Resource Based Relative Value Scale".
Member	The insured individual covered by the various health insurance products issued by Health Maintenance Organizations. Also known as the "Patient" or "Enrollee" (by Medicare).
MRI	Magnetic Resonance Imaging
MSA	Metropolitan Service Area – Geographically specified areas defined by Congress used to determine average Medicare/Medicaid costs and establish locally specific Medicare Fee Schedules.
NCQA	National Committee for Quality Assurance
NDC	National Drug Code—A national classification system for identifying drugs. Analogous to CPT codes for medical procedures.

Network	The network is the group of providers contracted with an insurance company or MCO to provide defined services at a contracted fee.
Palliative Care	Comfort care provided to relieve pain rather than pursue an improbable cure for a terminally ill patient.
Patient	The person considered an "Enrollee" by Medicare, an "Insured" by an Indemnity Company or a "Member" of an HMO.
Payor (payer)	The payor is the organization that transfers funds from the purchaser to the provider. Payors may be insurance companies, TPAs, ASOs, or MCOs.
PCP	Primary Care Provider—A physician practicing family medicine, pediatrics or ObGyn.
PPO	Preferred Provider Organization—A network of providers assembled by an insurance company to deliver health care to insureds at a negotiated fee schedule.
POEMR	Problem Oriented Electronic Medical Record. An EMR using a database that organizes information by the patient's problem rather than origin or source.
POMR	Problem Oriented Medical Record—Organization of patient information by problem rather than source of the data. May be paper or electronic.
POS	Point of Service—The place where medical decisions and made and medical care is delivered (e.g., provider's office, hospital, emergency room, etc.). The POS insurance option allows the insured to utilize out of network providers at a higher cost.
PRO	Professional Review Organization—A government administrative team of medical professionals employed to review physician practices.

Provider	The medical professional or institution that provides the medical services to the insured population covered by the various health insurance products. Synonymous with Physician or other medical personal administering a service to a patient (insured, enrollee, member).
Purchaser	The employer group or individual that has selected ("Purchased") one of the various health insurance products marketed by insurance companies, TPAs, ASOs and MCOs.
QA	Quality Assurance—Measuring and reporting the process of delivering health care to determine if evidence based medicine and sound business practices have been followed.
Quality Care	Quality care is appropriate, effective, efficient and accessible.
RWJ	Robert Wood Johnson Foundation—Largest U.S. philanthropic organization concerned with health care issues.
Rating	Underwriter determination of rates for insurance policies or health contracts for classes of risks.
Self-Funded	A self-funded health care plan is underwritten entirely by the employer. A self-funded plan may be self-administered, or employ a TPA or ASO to process claims. Self-funded plans obtain reinsurance (stop loss) to cover catastrophic claims.
Setting	The location where health care services are provided (example: inpatient facility, nursing home, etc.).
Single Payor System	The concept of one Insurance/claims processing company administering all payment for government purchased programs for all Americans.
Single Purchaser System	Taxpayer financed universal coverage with the government as the sole purchaser of services, administered by many private claims processors.

Specialist, secondary care	Physicians with medical or surgical specialty certification (e.g., internal medicine, general surgery, cardiology, orthopedics, ophthalmology, otolaryngology, dermatology, etc.).
Specialist, tertiary care	Physicians with advanced subspecialty certification (e.g., endocrinology, neurology, neurosurgery, neonatology, etc.).
TPA	Third Party Administrator—A claims processing company that adjudicates medical bills for covered employees working for a large, self funded employer. TPAs do not manage risk.
Underwriter	The indemnity insurance company employee who determines the risk of loss and selects the premium for the individual or employer group.
Underwriting	The process of risk selection, classification and evaluation, according to insurability. The process assures that the group covered has the same probability of loss as the population on which premium rates were based.
UR	Utilization Review—A managed care technique of applying criteria and standards of medical care prior to authorizing payment for requested medical services. Similar to utilization management (UM).
URO	Utilization Review Organization—Usually a freestanding organization of medical professionals that contract with an ASO or Insurance Company to provide Precertification.
Work-Up	A complete patient evaluation including laboratory tests, imaging studies, medical history, physical exam and diagnostic procedures.

References and Web Pages

www.rogerhstrubemd.com

www.creativedesignforhealthcarereform.us

Ashworth, Kenneth H. (2001). *Caught Between the Dog and the Fireplug, or, How to Survive Public Service.*

Bureau of Labor Statistics, www.bls.gov

Berns, Gregory. (2008) *Iconoclast: a neuroscientist reveals how to think differently,* Harvard Business School Publishing Corporation

Capra, Frank (Producer & Director). (1947). *It's a Wonderful Life* (Motion Picture). USA: Liberty Films II.

Centers for Medicare & Medicaid Services. "National Health Expenditure (NHE) Fact Sheet." http://www.cms.gov/NationalHealthExpendData/25_NHE_Fact_Sheet.asp#TopOfPage

Dartmouth Atlas, www.dartmouthatlas.org.

Daschle, Senator Tom with Scott S. Greenberger and Jeanne M. Lambrew. (2008). *Critical:* Dean, Howard. (2009) *Prescription for Real Healthcare Reform,* Chelsea Green Publishing. Vermont

Deming, W. Edwards. (1986). *Out of the Crisis.* Cambridge, MA: MIT Press.

"Effective Care." A Dartmouth Atlas Project Topic Brief. Page 2. Retrieved on January 18, 2011 from http://www.dartmouthatlas.org/downloads/reports/effective_care.pdf.

Dirksen, Senator. http://www.dirksencenter.org/print_emd_billionhere.htm

Filion, Kai. (2010, January 14). "Downcast Unemployment Forecast—Targeted Job Creation Policies Necessary to Offset Grim Projections." Economic Policy Institute.

http://www.deha.org/Glossary/GlossaryA.htm#top

http://www.epi.org/publications/entry/ib270/.

http://www.naifa.org/advocacy/health/documents/Comparing_HealthCare_Admin_Costs.pdf

http://www.nbc.com/saturday-night-live/recaps/#cat=10&mea=396&ima=92203

http://www-cgi.cnn.com/ALLPOLITICS/1996/news/9608/30/clinton.speech/clinton.shtml.

Interqual: http://www.mckesson.com.

Med 2005; 353:487-497

Madison, James (under the pseudonym "Publius"). (1787, November 23). "The Federalist No. 10." http://www.constitution.org/fed/federa10.htm

MarketWatch: "Illness And Injury As Contributors To Bankruptcy" by David U. Himmelstein,

Mary Walton and W. Edwards Deming, (1986). *The Deming Management Method.* NY: The Berkley Publishing Group.

Millenson, Michael. (1997) *Demanding Medical Excellence. Doctors and accountability in the information age.* The University of Chicago Press

Milliman & Roberson: http://www.milliman.com/home/index.php.

National Health Care Anti-Fraud Association. "Consumer Info & Action." http://www.nhcaa.org/eweb/DynamicPage.aspx?webcode=anti_fraud_resource_centr&wpscode=ConsumerAndActionInfo.

National Health Care Anti-Fraud Association. "Consumer Info & Action." http://www.nhcaa.org/eweb/DynamicPage.aspx?webcode=anti_fraud_resource_centr&wpscode=ConsumerAndActionInfo.

Osterberg, Lars M.D., and Terrence Blaschke, M.D. "Adherence to Medication." N Engl J

Regional and Racial Variation in Primary Care and the Quality of Care Among Medicare Beneficiaries http://www.dartmouthatlas.org/downloads/reports/Primary_care_report_090910.pdf

Regional and Racial Variation in Primary Care and the Quality of Care Among Medicare Beneficiaries http://www.dartmouthatlas.org/downloads/reports/Primary_care_report_090910.pdf

Secure Horizons Health Plan. https://www.securehorizons.com/

What we can do about the health-care crisis. NY: St. Martins Press.

Silver Sneakers: http://www.silversneakers.com/

Supply-Sensitive Care A Dartmouth Atlas Project Topic Brief http://www.dartmouthatlas.org/downloads/reports/supply_sensitive.pdf

The Animals. (1965, US). "Don't Let Me Be Misunderstood." MGM Records. Writers: Bennie Benjamin, Gloria, Caldwell, & Sol Marcus. Producer: Mickie Most. Retrieved on December 26, 2010 from http://en.wikipedia.org/wiki/Don%27t_Let_Me_Be_Misunderstood.

U.S. Health and Human Services. http://healthit.hhs.gov

US Bureau of Labor Statistics. (2010, September 10). Economic News Release: "Number of Jobs Held, Labor Market Activity, and Earnings Growth Among the Youngest Baby Boomers: Results From a Longitudinal Survey Summary." http://www.bls.gov/news.release/nlsoy.nr0.htm.

US Bureau of the Census. (2009). Table HIA-1. Health Insurance Coverage Status and Type of Coverage by Sex, Race and Hispanic Origin: 1999 to 2009. http://www.census.gov/hhes/www/hlthins/data/historical/index.html.

VanGiezen, Robert, and Albert E. Schwenk. (originally posted fall 2001). "Compensation from before World War I through the Great Depression." Bureau of Labor Statistics. http://www.bls.gov/opub/cwc/cm20030124ar03p1.htm.

Walton, Mary and Deming, W. Edwards. (1986). *The Deming Management Method.* NY: The Berkley Publishing Group.

Warren, Elizabeth, Deborah Thorne, and Steffie Woolhandler. (2 February 2005). http://content.healthaffairs.org/cgi/content/full/hlthaff.w5.63/DC1.

Weed, Lawrence L. (1969). *Medical Records, Medical Education, and Patient Care: The Problem-Oriented Record as a Basic Tool.* Cleveland: Press of Case Western Reserve University. http://lccn.loc.gov/69017686

Weed, Lawrence L. (1991). *Knowledge Coupling: New Premises and New Tools for Medical Care and Education.* N.Y. Springer-Verlag.

World Health Organization. (2000). "The World Health Report 2000—Health Systems: Improving Performance. http://www.who.int/whr/2000/en/index.html. See "Annex Table 1 Health system attainment and performance in all Member States, ranked by eight measures, estimates for 1997"

Index